WHY I RUN ?

AN EXHILARATING RUNNING SAGA OF ALPANA AGARWAL

NALIN RAI

Made with ♥ on the Notion Press Platform
www.notionpress.com

This work would not have seen the light of day without the support of my family including my wife Suman, daughter Sneha and son Vinayak who continue to endure with me and bear my idiosyncrasies and the mood swings that the writers are associated with.

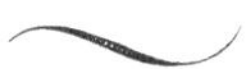

Of course, were it not for Alpana who kept on remembering one thing or the other as the draft progressed, this work would not have gravitated towards a finality as it did. Alpana thank you for agreeing to share your story with the world out there.

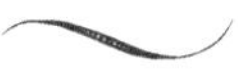

Above all, to all the women who are fighting their battles to keep fit and keep their weight under control, don't lose heart, if Alpana could do it, then you also can.

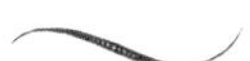

Contents

Foreword

"The man who moves a mountain begins by carrying away small stones." – <u>Confucius</u>

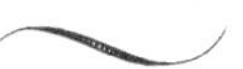

It was a chance encounter during the Alumni meet of Kendriya Vidyalaya Tagore Garden, New Delhi with Alpana Agarwal in 2014 where she shared the fact that she was a runner. We had been in the same class but in different sections, but the class solidarity caught on and I started keeping a tab on the running sojourn of Alpana. Social Media was a great facilitating device for keeping a tab on her activity.

Her association with running was gaining momentum. When she completed her First Half Marathon, the Standard Chartered Mumbai Marathon, the writer in me saw a story unspooling and a story that needed to be told to the world. The story had the punchline or the meat as we writers say, and it started evolving. As Alpana celebrated her 55th birthday in August 2022 and completed her 55th long-distance run, the story also reached its finishing line or the podium finish as the runners say.

The exciting part of the story is that this is a story of grit, resolve and commitment without any family background associated with the run. Whatever she has achieved in her running career has been her indulgence and commitment without any regular trainer. Her motivation was Fauja Singh and she wishes to emulate his footsteps by continuing to run until she dies. Well, when she does complete 108 races, maybe it would be time to do a 2.0 of this version. For the time being, readers, enjoy this journey, more so the women readers as it is a story that inspires. The unfolding of the story has also taken a long time, akin to the time Alpana took to become an accomplished runner!

Etymologically Alpana in Hindi means **rangoli** or floor art which is the domain of women in India per se. It is an art that demands concentration, focus, and the ability to envisage colours in myriad combinations and to weave them into a construct that just mesmerizes the viewer. After all, the medium used is powdered colour and each of the demarcations of colour are so neatly arranged that the feeling captivates.

Alpana's journey has been akin to making a Rangoli which on a path of evolution and adaptation starts with a monochrome colour, an analogy from Alpana's journey of Marathon in the form of initial reluctance and then bursting on in the form of a riot of colours manifest in testing the mettle in different kinds of races and coming out as a winner with flying colours. The analogy of Rangoli with the saga of run that Alpana has traversed in his life so far has been used as Alpana has traversed this journey on her own without any coach, guide or mentor. It is a self-taught quest which rumbles through experiments and quests, permeated with oodles of self-belief and energy e.g. her experimentation to mark the distance for running by traversing the distance through her scooter and then using it for preparation of her races.

Rangoli is a manifestation of happiness, positivity and liveliness of a household and this is what Alpana's running saga has been about. She derives happiness from running the race and not hankering for the time or chasing records, it has brought an element of positivity in her life and the positivity in the household from her running saga is manifest from the fact that her husband as also her children derive pleasure in running along with her. She would derive her ultimate happiness when her husband runs along with her for a full Marathon and I would be waiting for it in gleeful anticipation as once that happens the final topping of Rangoli would be achieved.

Happy Reading

Nalin Rai

Preface

I found the marvellous real with every step.
Alejo Carpentier

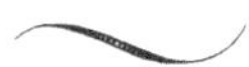

Acknowledgements

Wikipedia, Distance Running Magazine-UK, History.com, Forrest Gump (1994), Sole2Soul.com, Pintrest.com, Garret Kramer- Stillpower- Excellence with ease in Sports and Life (2011), Centre for Enhancement of Learning & Teaching of Pirfysgol Bangor University-London

Pictures: Seema Chaubey

Prologue

"The miracle isn't that I finished.
The miracle is that I had the courage to start." – **John Bingham**

When we conjure up the nomenclature **running**, what is the image immediately registered through our visual cortex? The image that immediately pops up in mind is of a runner laden with sweat dripping body-blissfully unaware of the unending outflow of the sweat. Focused attention towards a target that is hanging like a low-hanging fruit in not too a distant vision, enticing and inspiring to go for. An ultimate expression of endurance that the human form can aspire. It is sublime in manifestation and rawest in exposition-! The podium beckoned to scale it.

Obviously, this image has a masculine representation across civilizations and seldom does one find feminine imagery associated with this process. Man has always been a runner, since the advent of civilization and it is a natural expression of his composition! He was a hunter – running was one of the basic things, which he adopted to excel in the art of hunting as also as a part of his survival streak. In fact, the common person stopped running just for the last few hundred years.

With health consciousness creeping in and the lifestyles that have become the norm, running established itself as a process to reconnect with nature, or has it shifted indoors in quite a lot of cases in an air-conditioned environment?

Men were running, but now women also have started hitting the asphalt energetically or the automated tracks of the gym, competing for a shoulder to shoulder with their male brethren to carve a space for themselves in the space of running as well.

This saga is of one such woman who took up running, and it has now become her brand identity and her raison d'tre (reason of existence). The saga unfolded by the urge to lose weight and to return to the pink of health.

An average Indian middle-class woman generally is seen walking in a group with women or spouses (a rare sight) or with their children; it is conventionally more of a group activity, social interaction and updating event- a sort of message and gossip circulation about the habitats where they reside. A woman running lonely on the roads still is a sighting that veneers to irregularity in its appearance, though it has started acquiring a sporadic manifestation with regularity in the metropolitan cities of the country.

This story is a story of shedding inhibitions about running on the Indian roads and the saga began when Alpana Agarwal- yes, time to introduce the woman or the character of the book whose transformation through a marathon is the story that has been chronicled as a compilation of inspiration for others to follow suit.

It started taking shape when Alpana landed in Mumbai subsequent to the transfer of her husband in 2012. By profession, Alpana is a teacher. When was the last time one has seen a schoolteacher running? She is sapped handling the new generation and moulding them in a positive manner on a daily basis by the time the day concludes! Being a schoolteacher, one seldom associates them with running and Alpana was in the same league until she decided to break from it, though the unshackling took some time to happen.

When, or the first time an opportunity was presented to her to participate in a 5km run as a part of annual day celebrations at the Navy Children School in Delhi, she could not tear herself away from the household responsibilities and found it difficult to start early in the morning for the run.

However, both her sons got themselves baptized on the occasion into the art of running and went for the run consecutively for two years while the family was posted in Delhi. However, for the woman in question, running still was a dreadful nightmare! She could never visualize herself slipping into running gear early in the morning and zooming on for a 5km trip... and when she rewinds and reminisces the reluctance and Alpana of the present times, both are like an anti-thesis to each other as she underlined the evolution with a twinkle of her eye. Those were the days...

CHAPTER ONE

THE PROCESS AND THE MOTIVATION

"Running is the greatest metaphor for life because you get out of it what you put into it."— Oprah Winfrey

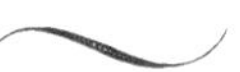

Centre for enhancement of Learning & Teaching of Prifysgol Bangor University, London has defined the characteristics of runners as:

1. Determination
2. Resilience
3. Flexibility
4. Self-belief
5. Growth mindset
6. Good time Management

In addition, the icing on the cake of the characteristics of runners defined by the University is that:

"**They Are Not Normal**".

Indeed, Alpana started her running sojourn, perhaps inspired by the Quotation- "**They are not normal!**" which she may not have been aware of at all when she decided to start running! After all, without a history of running in the family or inspiration from near and dear ones to run- how does one start running one fine day? A Forest Gump did start, but he was of the male variety!

For Alpana, it was an internal process, it evolved over a period, and riding on the bandwagon of self-confidence and self-belief catapulted her into a Marathon runner. The journey was exhilarating as the green shoots started appearing when she was approaching her mid-forties!

They say about Mumbai that the city grows on you and it inspires you to try out something new, which you may not have done in your life at all before landing in Mumbai! It happened with Alpana as well. The green shoots of running for Alpana began when she shifted to Mumbai in November 2011 after the transfer of her husband (A Naval Officer).

Mumbai had firmly ensconced itself as the running capital of India after the advent the of Standard Chartered Mumbai Marathon in 2004. It kindled the spirit of running in the Mumbaikars- interspersed with profuse dollops of celebrities as a glam quotient in the initial stages. Alpana was also bitten by the bug of visible manifestation in the form of runners sprinting around the locality she stayed (Navy Nagar in Colaba where she was putting up - is a dream location for runners and one can find runners running along the serene surrounding of the colony as also alongside the Arabian Sea).

A proud mother of two sons and wife of a Naval Officer regular walks have been a part of her upbringing as it was the template in most of the middle-class families of the times of the seventies and eighties when children used to walk to the neighbourhood. Her running sojourn is also an outcome of the mid-life crisis that most of us face-the weight gain around 45 years or so. It is the genie uncorked which refuses to go back into the bottle, i.e. slim and trim figure! (In addition, this mid-life crisis is gender neutral). She tried all tricks under the sun but her weight refused to budge on the downslide at all!

For Alpana, it all began the running that is, as a desperate attempt to knock off a few inches and kilos and bring down the number that popped up and shocked her every time she stood on the weighing scales. Perhaps Mumbai did the trick for her to shed her inhibitions and stay focused on the job at hand- (the **determination part of the characteristic** to knock off the few kilos).

When she started running, the process was an admixture of shyness of running garnished with a self-fixed target- to shed down the weight.

In the initial stages she would just screech to a halt if she found somebody crossing her path while she was running (the burden of embarrassment applying the brakes), but now she does not even take cognizance of her husband if he crossed her path while she was running her race! Mumbai was the catalytic confidence booster for her!

Her embarrassment of running when she encountered somebody crossing her path was replaced with a determination to make a success out of it when she read about the story of Fauja Singh- the famous marathon runner who started running again at the ripe old age of 89 years!

He became the inspiration that Alpana had been searching for as the motivation to hit the turf! If Fauja Singh could start running again at 89 years of age to get rid of the hurt and pain of the passing away of his wife- Alpana was half of his age! She was fighting her internal demons, they had to be annihilated, and what better way to do that than to sweat it out and let them disappear along with the sweat?

Therefore, the quest began! Alpana still succinctly remembers the date- it was 01 March 2012, when she decided to switch over from daily walking to jogging. The initial jog for a few meters did hesitatingly soon become a daily ritual. Slowly-slowly, the confidence started building up and she achieved a circuit of four km. It became the rigour- and the results were visible within three months.

The extra kilos just melted away. Alpana was back in shape and started getting compliments on her new looks – a direct outcome of sweat and glory. Running changed her persona and she became a very positive person, and her patience levels increased. It has become a rigour as when she runs she gets rid of all her stress and negativity pouring out along with sweat leaving her with glowing skin which no gold or pearl facial can provide.

She ran her first half Marathon in February 2015 at the age of 47 yrs. and 6 months, the green shoots sprouting out after three years. She still has goosebumps about what she has achieved.

With a sense of pride, she remembers: "When I run I am oblivious to the entire world. I feel one with nature. I just concentrate on my run and I am so lost in my thoughts that I do not pay any attention to passersby on the road. Many times, it happens that known faces greet me when I am running but I just see through them without a hint of recognition. I have given lost looks even

to my husband and kids when they crossed me on my run!

One would not know whether runners running around different parts of the country and in different nooks and corners of the world face the same dilemma of acknowledging known faces while running, but Alpana did face it persistently. It indeed is comical, to say the least, that when a runner is focused on the job at hand (to finish the run), how could she or he acknowledge a known face which loomed into the horizon and then ebbed away- and Alpana has not even bothered to acknowledge her husband while running, what to talk of other known faces! She has faced the comments of the known faces - but along with Alpana, her family has taken it in their stride with pride!

Relatives, spouses, and well-wishers need to understand that for a runner it is a herculean task **to run and acknowledge greetings simultaneously. When the runner hits the tarmac and as the shoes pound the asphalt below, with each thrust the creative urge keeps on manifesting, and with each step as the focus gets accentuated, several decisions hanging in limbo reach their finality. It is a stage of sublime submergence with the soul and serenity.**

Alpana has another reason for not acknowledging anybody while running. She is myopic! Moreover, while running she does not wear her glasses! The result is, while running, she can't see clearly who is coming from the opposite direction until the person comes closer and on top of that she is engrossed in her world of thoughts- as a result even known faces appear as a blip on her screen.

After all, while running her mind is more focused on a nutritious meal to make up for the energy loss that she has to endure. The rush of adrenalin of creative urges also manifests to its acme and she narrated an instance to substantiate it:

"When we were in Delhi in 2011, a senior Naval Officer was retiring and a get-together was organized to bid farewell to his wife. On that occasion, organizers invited entries for a poem on farewell. The winner of the best poem apart from the winning prize had also to recite it. I also submitted my poem that took shape while running and then went away for a preplanned vacation to Kashmir. On our return, I came to know that my poem got the best poem award. However, as I was not there my friend read it out and received the prize on my behalf. Here is the poem...

Farewell, my dear,
May the sun shine brighter
Your load be lighter
Into a new realm
May you find peace and calm.
Farewell, my dear,
May flowers bloom
And take away your gloom
To bring joy and happiness
And shower upon you God's kindness,
Farewell, my dear,
Your journey has just begun
Be hopeful, don't be glum
Leave your worries and sorrows
And embrace the smiling tomorrow.
Farewell, my dear,
May your dreams come true
Our best wishes are with you
Whenever you need us
We shall be there for you.

Alpana writes for the in-house Naval annual magazine "Veerangana" which is published for the naval personnel and their families. The ideas to write on the given theme generally evolve during her walks/runs. She encapsulates:

I cannot believe where I have reached today when I compare the reluctance to run with my family at children's school! During those initial days of running, I had never thought even in the wildest of my dreams that one day I will run not only marathons but an ultra-marathon as well. Several times, I try to open the closed doors of my mind and rake the childhood memories to see if I had shown any inclination towards running or any other similar activity. However, to my dismay nothing turns up, it is a dark zone. I only remember various outdoor games that we as children used to play in the 70s and early 80s. These games like kho- kho, langdi tang, chain, and many others involved running but then I am sure I was not an exceptional runner in these games.

Faint memories of the spoon and lemon race, sack race and three-legged race in my childhood also turn up but here also I fared as an average participant. I also used to play basketball in my school days but I fail to conjure up anything in particular that would throw some light on my running capability, which had suddenly surfaced in the latter half of my life.

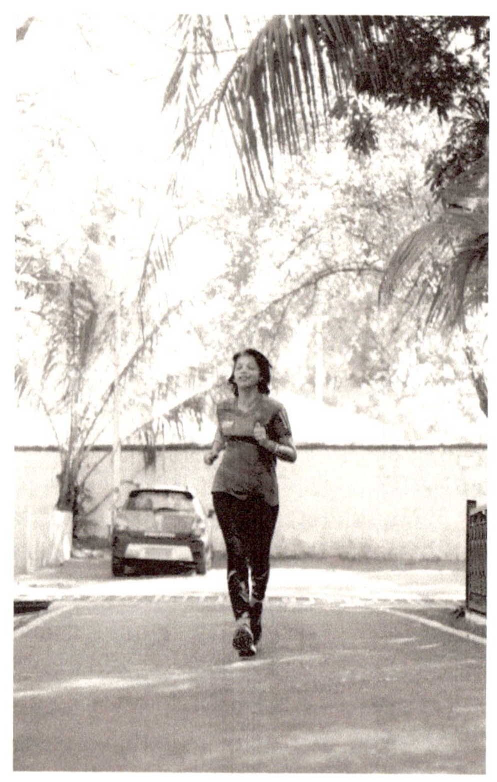

CHAPTER TWO

RUN BEGINS PROFESSIONALLY

"If you don't have answers to your problems after a four-hour run, you ain't getting them." –
Christopher McDougall

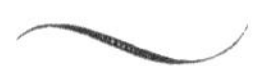

How many people in India do you think would run 5km, 10 km, 21 km or 42 km, just for fun? Quite a few. The first major running event in India was held in 2004 in Mumbai, the Standard Chartered Mumbai Marathon, though Pune led back in 1998. In 2015, we had nearly 150 running events across the country. Today, this figure must have crossed 500 easily. In Mumbai alone, there is a running event somewhere in the city almost every Sunday.

Tata Mumbai Marathon (yes, after Tatas took it over, now it is known as Tata Mumbai Marathon), is a marque event for the country. For the year 2023, there were 7201 finishers. A total of 10993 finished the Half Marathon. In 2022 Women finishers in both categories, Half Marathon and Full Marathon improved from the last event (pre-Covid) with 9% of total finishers in Marathon and about

19% of finishers in Half-Marathon. (So, the introductory premise that women still are in lesser numbers in long-distance running holds good and the numbers need to increase). Besides these numbers are with a negative split. (source:geeksonfeet.com)

Mumbai Marathon is among the top ten marathons in the world in terms of its classification. It is the World Athletics Gold Label Road Race event. Distance running or endurance running is a form of continuous running over distances of at least 8 km. There are four main types of runs-10 km, Half Marathon – 21.1 km, Full Marathon – 42.2 km, and Ultra Marathon – any distance greater than 42.2 km.

All the races have varied age categories in both male and female gender separately. The minimum age to run a Marathon is generally 18 years, though even 12-year-old contestants can run up to 5km or 10 km., as per the rules laid down by the organizers. Every year hundreds of runners participate in these running events. Significantly, women across all age groups and profiles are signing up for races. Indian women are breaking barriers and stepping out of their comfort zones to participate in these running events.

Marathon finish is classified with two kinds of splits- a positive split and a negative split. It is observed among the runners that the second half of racing is slower than the first half. It is known as positive split and is characterized by increased oxygen consumption, higher level of fatigue and increased rate of perceived exertion (RPE). A negative split on the other is characterized by the ability to complete the second half of the Marathon at a faster pace than the first half of the Marathon. Mumbai Marathon has a 96% positive split, and a 4% negative split (source:geeksonfeet.com).

For Alpana, her baptism into running started taking shape in 2013, when she embarked on the process to complete running inside the vast expanse of the Navy Nagar complex, in Colaba, Mumbai.

It however presented her with a peculiar situation where her running time clashed with her husband's (Ajay) coming home from the office. She had told Ajay to carry a spare set of keys. As Ajay was not used to the habit of carrying spare keys, when he returned home in the evening, he would find a locked house mocking his forgetfulness.

He would then ring up to inform Alpana that he is waiting but seldom came an occasion where Alpana gave up her running to run back to attend to her husband, she would come to the house only after finishing the chore for the day, i.e. completing her run!

Her husband never cribbed and waited patiently with a smiling face. He has been a pillar of strength and the backroom boy to help Alpana run her marathon races of different hues, and the process of forgetting the keys of the house was his default mechanism to welcome Alpana when she came back after her running.

The First Professional Run

Alpana's marathon journey may not have even taken off, if her husband had not informed her about the 10 km spirit run being held in March 2013 on Women's Day-DNA I CAN. DNA, the newspaper published from Mumbai, organized DNA I Can.

She was quite happy and satisfied with her routine run of 4-5 km in the evenings. Her husband, a few days before the **DNA I Can** Mumbai Run, informed her about this event and suggested that she should now test the water by registering for it.

Alpana was shell-shocked that her husband aspired that she should run a 10 km event! Her first reaction was "**NO, I can't do it**". However, he kept on motivating her and even advised her to walk if she found it difficult to run but not to run away from it before trying it out. His persistence finally paid off and Alpana agreed to jump into the arena of professional running. Her husband who took the responsibility of online registration for the event started back-office work of running for Alpana with this run.

When she broke the news to her friends about her participation in the 10 km run, they were also thrilled. After all, Alpana was the first among her friends who had decided to test her mettle in the arena of professional running on the wrong side of the forties.

When the D-Day of debut run arrived, confidence was gushing in her veins with determination to prove to the world that one more runner was ready to make her debut in long-distance running and it was going to be a long-term love affair with the tracks!

The 10 km run was to start at 6 AM and she reached the venue at around 5.30 AM. She joined the warm-up Zumba sessions as her preparation for the run and waited expectantly for the first long-distance run of her life. Though a bit apprehensive, with butterflies in her stomach, the only thing she was confident about was that come what may she would finish the run.

Once the run started, her strong willpower and utter elation of being in the process of professional running continued to be her companion on a roller coaster ride and she did not stop even once, not even for a water break, during the entire run of 10 km. The **determination-another characteristic of the marathon runner** -became her sounding board to complete the event!

The initial few meters were a bit uncomfortable as she was used to running on the track during her practice runs and here she was running on a concrete road! Soon she got the hang of the concrete road catalyzed by her husband cheered her along the route. Though the run was only for women, he ran along with her for the last few meters, much to the chagrin of the organizers and to the delight of the onlookers who cheered them with amused looks on their faces.

Having completed her first 10 km run, the sense of accomplishment in the form of an effervescent smile never left her face. As she collected her Medal and snack box after the run, she ran into an old acquaintance who told Alpana that she ran 21 km.

ALPANA AGARWAL
Yes You Can!

This is to certify that you have successfully participated in
Stayfree Women For Change DNA iCan Women's Half Marathon
on
10th March 2013
in the
Spirit Run (10 km)

Certificate of First Marathon Run (Half Marathon)

Alpana froze in her steps! She wondered if she would ever run 21km in her lifetime. She calculated that to reach the venue for a 10km run she had to get up at 4 AM, so for running 21km, she would have to get up at 3 AM and start from her place at 4 AM as the run started at 5.30 AM. The mere thought of waking up at this unearthly hour for a run sounded weird and immediately she threw such absurd thoughts out of her mind. Instead, she focused on revelling in the excitement of successfully finishing her first 10km and proudly adorned her finisher's medal. Who knew...that a few years later getting up at 3 AM would become a regular affair for Alpana!

While she was basking in the glory of her first triumph, in the background a new situation was unfolding!

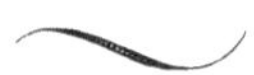

CHAPTER THREE

CHANGE OF BASE TO MHOW

"If you run, you are a runner. It does not matter how fast or how far.

It does not matter if today is your first day or if you have been running for twenty years.

There is no test to pass, no license to earn, no membership card to get. You just run." – **John Bingham**

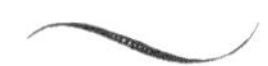

In 2013, Alpana's husband informed her that he stands transferred from Mumbai to Mhow (a cantonment in the Indore district, in Madhya Pradesh). There was resistance in the family against shifting base, more so from Alpana. There is a famous saying for Mumbai- one who arrives in this city, seldom leaves it for good, and by hook or crook buys a roof over their head.

Alpana had the lurking fear in her mind that she may not have the same kind of running facilities in Mhow as she had in Mumbai and to which she had become quite accustomed- and which her husband had underlined as a transition quotient for smooth shifting. Her husband ensured that Mhow had all the required facilities and she would not miss Mumbai.

Shift to Mhow eventually happened but the first brush with the geography at Mhow was a shocker, to say the least for Alpana and her children! The difference between Mumbai, a metro, and Mhow, a small city, stared in the face! After having lived in one of the most enviable postal codes of the country - Colaba- Alpana felt she has shifted to Nayagaon (a distant suburb on the Western Local Railway line in Mumbai) when she landed in Mhow. While going through the process of settling down in Mhow, Alpana's worst fears came true! Mhow did not have any dedicated jogging/ running track!

Upset at her husband supposedly not being aware of the ground realities of Mhow, Alpana confronted him on his statement about Mhow having a running track. Using his charm, the husband however was able to calm her down by saying that for a long-distance runner, the road is the companion and Road was in existence in diversified forms of manifestations in Mhow as well! Besides, being a marathon runner, practising on the road was a better option than running on the racing tracks! Alpana veneered around to her husband's viewpoint and started running on the tiled pavements of Mall road and other adjoining roads in Mhow.

Mhow being a small place, the sight of a woman running on the road, all alone, in a civil area was a rarity. People on the roads would give her a second look whenever Alpana would loom on their horizon pounding the tracks. However, she was unruffled by their reaction and continued with her practice. Her perseverance bore fruit.

Soon, stares turned into smiles and some regular walkers whom she used to cross almost daily even started saying Hello! This change in the attitude of the common public delighted her. Soon her friends and colleagues started cracking jokes about her running ritual. They commented that she would have to bear the cost of wear and tear on the roads arising out of sustained pounding on the asphalt.

IIM Indore Run

As she became acclimatized to her new training ground at Mhow, Alpana came to know that IIM Indore was organizing an 11km run on 2 Oct 2013.

She was accompanied by her husband on the day of the event, who was condescending enough to miss his weekly round of Golf (a big sacrifice. really!). It had rained heavily the previous night and Alpana was not sure if the event would be held at all!

Hoping for the best she went ahead and reached the venue much before the starting time. After a quick warm-up session, it was time to line up at the start line. Soon, the run started and she kept surging ahead. All along the route, there were several temples, and as she crossed them one by one, she prayed to each one of the Gods residing in those abodes to give her the strength and stamina to complete the run.

The route had some undulating terrain but undeterred by the upslope, she continued running. Her prayers were answered that day and despite the challenging route, she did manage to finish the run in good time.

As she crossed the finish line, the organizers informed her that she had secured first place in her age group of 45 years + female category. She just could not believe this and cross-checked once again. The organizers assured her that she indeed was the winner! She felt like dancing and shouting out to the world. She immediately called home and informed her children and her other family members about her podium finish.

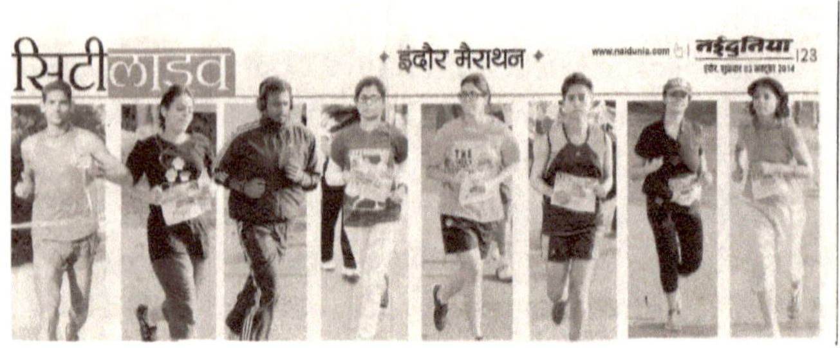

Indore Marathon

Though she had to wait for some time for the prize ceremony, for Alpana winner's trophy in her hands was all that mattered to her. It was an incredible achievement as Alpana was running her second major race and emerged at the top. She reminisced: "The euphoria and elation that rushed through me were incredible, the sheer joy of holding the trophy was an experience which I had not gone through in my life after the birth of my children"!

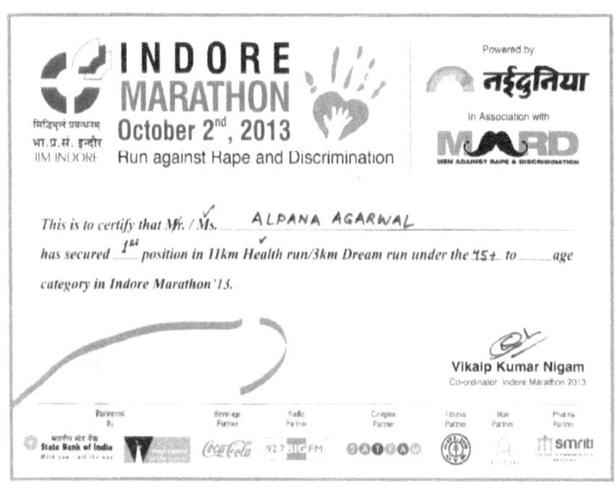

Indore Marathon Certificate

When October 2014 opened itself, she was there again on the track to do an encore in the 11km run organized by IIM Indore. Same venue and same route and she was better prepared this time. However, the organizers had different plans! They had altered the bar of the age category!

For 2014, the organizers of IIM Indore carved out a new category of 40-50 years. Now she had to compete with women five years younger than her, but still, she got the second position. It was a creditable performance by Alpana as the woman who won the first prize had just turned forty and had been running for a long time!

While chitchatting, waiting for the prize distribution trophy the champion revealed to Alpana that she was a member of the Indore runner's group and they travelled to different parts of India to participate in marathons. Alpana met the group leader and the group leader informed her that they were planning to run in the first Indore half Marathon in February next year. The leader of the runners' group was impressed with Alpana's running skills and encouraged her to target Half-Marathon. Alpana had a new scale to the summit- the Half Marathon.

The next day for the first time when she saw her pictures in the newspaper along with her feat of being included in the list of podium finishers, she knew that now she had earned the laurels to become a member of the long-distance running club. Alpana was now synonymous with a long-distance runner for friends and colleagues in Mhow. So, when on the occasion of 'INFANTRY DAY 'a 10 km run was organized at Mhow, it was taken for granted that Alpana would be a confirmed runner. She did arrive at the venue to find out that for the women the distance to be covered was only 3km!

She felt it was too timid a target to scale, but as it was for the sake of the fraternity, she decided to associate with it! A long-distance runner tries to find ways to walk the talk i.e. try and run the distance which is equivalent to a long-distance run on reaching the venue, Alpana finds some friends for the run, motivating them to do 10 km and luckily they too agreed.

The organizers were surprised that the participants had altered their plan but seeing the enthusiasm of the female runners to run 10 km, they acquiesced. It all began as a friendly run, but getting the tailwind, Alpana soon left her friends behind. Alpana finished the run in 64 minutes, leaving many *fauzi (army)* participants scampering for their breath to match up to her speed!

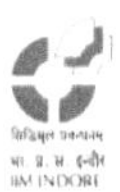
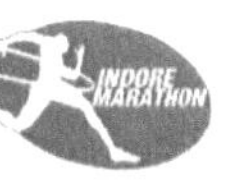

INDORE MARATHON 2014

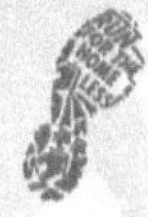
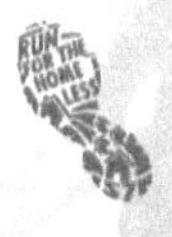

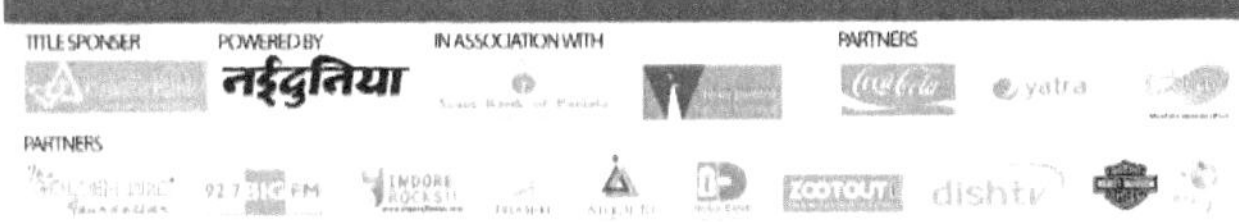

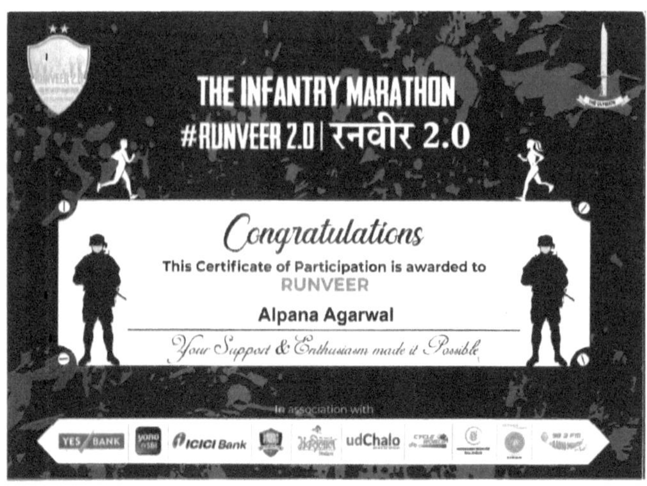

Infantry Marathon

CHAPTER FOUR

HALF MARATHON

"Running is alone time that lets my brain unspool the tangles
that build up over days...I run,
pound it out on the pavement, channel that energy into my
legs,
*and when I'm done with my run, I'm done with it." — **Rob***
Haneisen

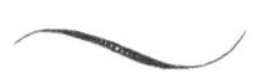

The fellow runners at the second leg of the IIM Indore Marathon convinced Alpana that she could run Half-Marathon and she started preparing for it mentally and physically. Though Alpana was confident of her running capabilities, Ajay was a bit sceptical. - He did not seem too excited about this new run! He was apprehensive that Alpana might not be able to cope with so much running in such a short period.

Nevertheless, through the **resilience** that had become a part of her DNA after she started running (**one of the core characteristics of the runner**), she persevered along. Seeing the commitment Ajay also veneered around to her determination and advised her to prepare systematically as she had to run 21 km for Indore Half Marathon in Feb.

2015.

5 months were available to Alpana before she could participate in the half marathon and she started preparing for it in right earnest. The biggest challenge was to gauge the distance of 21 km exactly, i.e. how to mark the coordinates, prepare the roadmap and start the preparation.

Smartwatches had started making their debut but Alpana was still oblivious to their existence. As a nation of JUGAAD, we work around things and Alpana was no exception- she decided to use her scooter to get around the problem.

She would ride her scooter and calculate the distance with the help of its speedometer. Though not accurate, it gave her an approximate idea of the distance to run daily to become eligible for a half-marathon. After marking the coordinates and flagging the route, she started by running small distances and slowly increased it by 2 km every week.

The maximum distance covered by her during the practice was 13-14 km. During practice runs, she frequently used to tumble on the road and would scrap her knees badly. However, the bruises were the stripes she earned by pounding the asphalt. Bruises as adornment steeled her commitment for the final day as it started looming on the horizon.

This being Central India's first major Half Marathon, grand-scale preparations were made to welcome national and international participants. There was a big crowd of runners full of *josh or the rush of adrenalin.* Some international marathoners were also participating in the event. Men and women alike were warming up for the run. The run started at sharp 5.30 AM and as the runners came out, they were showered with flower petals.

At some road junctions, there was even music blaring out from the speakers. One entire stretch was lined up with *bandwaalas (band players who play music on festive occasions in different parts of the country incorporating local adaptations)* playing popular feet-tapping music. People had lined up on both sides of the road to cheer and motivate the runners. As an encouragement to runners, they were adorned with Confetti. The entire city of Indore seemed to be out on the sidelines of the designated racetrack to cheer the participants who had taken a call to be a part of the inaugural Indore Half Marathon. Elaborate provision was made for water stations all along the race route. Music and dhol beats energized the runners. The whole atmosphere was that of festivity, fun and frolic.

The weather was perfect and Alpana was cruising along when after an hour or so, she found that there was a sudden groundswell in the number of runners. The sudden increase in the number of runners was because the participants who were running the 10 km marathon also merged in with the racers like Alpana, participants of the Half Marathon!

In that melee, she missed a crucial turn, which was the point of departure only for the half marathoners. In front of her was the vast expanse of 10km runners, as was evident from their bib numbers and she continued running along with them without realizing that 21km runners had to take a slightly different route. Subsequently, she missed the turn for the half-marathon and followed the runners ahead of her.

Once the runner missed the designated turn, the half-marathon distance was truncated to 18 km and Alpana did not realize it in the melee. Exalted at having braced the finishing line she was grinning from ear to ear after receiving her Finisher's medal. As she met other runners and started chatting with them, she noticed some of them were upset and grumbling about missing a turn. She was basking in the glory of her achievement and did not pay much attention to their grumbling, as she was sure she had run the entire distance of 21.1 km.

On the way back home, the grumbling unspooled in Alpana's mind as well. Her unease was compounded by the fact that she did not receive any message from the organizers about the time that she had clocked in to finish the supposed half-marathon and that her name did not figure in the finishers list as well!

Then it dawned on her that wily nilly she had also been a part of the grumbling of the fellow runners and she had run only 18 km as well! When a runner misses a turn on the route, she also misses the timing mat, which registers the time and distance covered by the runners as they step on it.

Organizers of the Marathon provide a bib number to all marathon runners and they have to compulsory pin it up on the front side of their t-shirts. The timed races have a timing chip inserted at the backside of the bib. All along the route, timing mats are placed at a specified distance and they record the timing as runners step on them so that their time is registered. If a runner misses a single mat, she is classified as **DNF. I.e. did not finish.**

As she reminisces with some sadness: "When this realization dawned on me I was thunderstruck. I could not believe that I had messed up my first half-marathon. It was gut-wrenching to know all that practice, sweat and scraped knees had been for nothing. I felt so guilty about missing this excellent opportunity of completing my first half marathon. I promised myself that I would run and complete the next half marathon that comes my way."

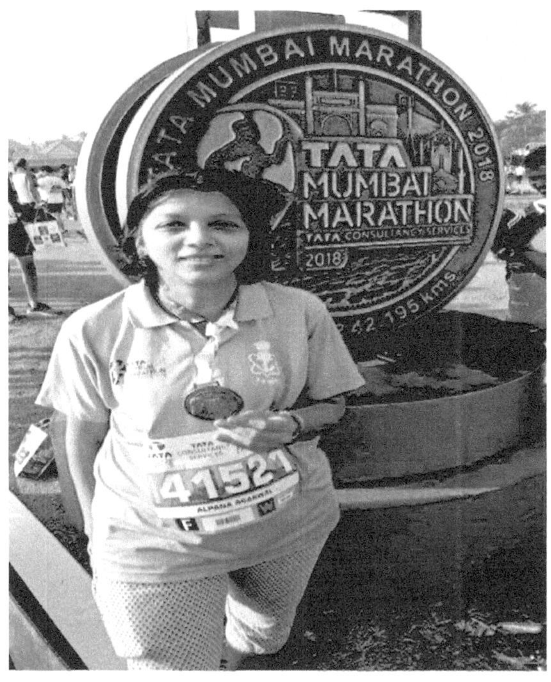

With the finisher Medal

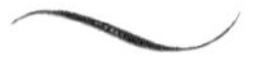

CHAPTER FIVE

BACK TO MUMBAI

"Don't fear moving slowly forward... fear standing still." –
Kathleen Harris

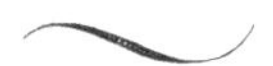

By May 2015, Alpana was back again in Mumbai after the transfer of her husband after a two-year tenure at Mhow. The scar of not having completed the half-Marathon was a soul tormentor that haunted her. To get rid of it, she slipped into practice mode, waiting for the opportunity to redeem herself.

She adopted the same method of marking her route and the distance with her scooter that she had done earlier when she had made her debut as a Marathon runner. In August 2015, as the Standard Chartered Mumbai Marathon for January 2016 was announced she was amongst the first to register for it. Once bitten twice shy, she exercised abundant caution in studying the route map and committing it to the memory.

As D-day arrived, the feeling of apprehension crept into her as she travelled down memory lane to share the feeling of D-Day. Star point was flooded with a huge swarm of runners. She was on the edge. However, with the firing of the gun at the starting point, she took off the block with confident strides. With the legs gaining momentum riding on the cheers of the spectators matching node to node with the beating of the drums creating an ambience of a motivating orchestra; she got a new spirit to her adrenalin.

With pride, she remembers: "I was running at a comfortable speed and enjoying my surroundings. The josh (rush of adrenalin) was at its peak and I pleasantly surprised myself by scaling the finish line without walking at all. That was my best time ever. I had clocked the distance of 21.1 km in 2 hours and 28 min. With great pride, I received my finishers' medal."

Alpana had redeemed herself and had fulfilled the commitment made to herself. The determination and the willpower to scale the target warded off the tiredness from making any inroads into her system. She stood 37/234 in the Mumbai Standard Chartered Marathon 2016 amongst the finishers in her gender and age category of 45 – 50 yrs.

At that point in time she had not planned any further summits to scale as she had decided first to finish off just one-half marathon. However, how naïve the thought was!

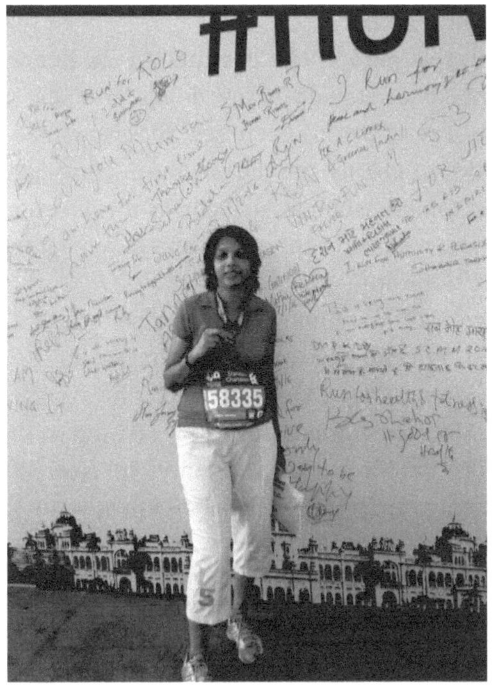

Stanchart Mumbi Marathon

Marathons galore

Now Alpana had entered the **Growth management characteristic** of the runners without realizing it- from one marathon to another. After graduating from one marathon to another, she came to know about the Navy Half Marathon. The western Naval Command in Mumbai was organizing a half marathon in Nov. 2016 and being from the Naval Community she wanted to be a part of this Marathon. She registered for the 21.1 km run and her younger son registered for the 10 km run. Her son performed quite well despite this being his first long-distance run. The Navy Half

Marathon happened in Nov.2016, and she ran this after a gap of eight months.

During this period, she continued with her walks and concentrated on staying fit by doing aerobics, yoga and other core strengthening exercises. She also joined the local gym inside her colony and did weight-bearing exercises. In July once, the monsoon started and as the weather became pleasant she resumed running and prepared herself for the next Half Marathon.

So, two Half Marathons were done and dusted in 2016. In Jan. 2017, again she ran 21.1km in Standard Chartered Mumbai Marathon. In October 2017, she ran 21.1 km in Customs Half Marathon followed by 21.1 km in the second edition of the Navy Half Marathon in Nov. 2017. Her husband Ajay ran his first official 10 km in Navy Marathon 2017.

While she was being baptized into the paraphernalia of professional running, she was still unaware of the different marathons held regularly in the city. So post her next Standard Chartered Mumbai Half Marathon in January 2018 she decided to take a break from running and concentrated on other ways of staying fit like aerobics, yoga etc.

It was during this period of break she met Blossom in Mumbai-an ultra-runner and a wonderful human being. They had an organic link through their sons who had studied together in school and were classmates, but the runner mothers did not know much about each other and hardly interacted. Alpana's son Shikhar however had informed her that Blossom too was a Marathon Runner.

In Sept. 2016, at a get- together many friends were talking about Blossom running a distance of 60km and even her son told Alpana that indeed Blossom had run a 60 km run. For Alpana, the fact was not sinking in!

Curiosity was getting her salivating in nervous excitement and when she met Blossom the next day at the vegetable market (yes runners like Alpana are normal housewives as well who perform the awesome task of running the household as also burning the asphalt in a Marathon) she congratulated her for being the talk of the town. Blossom convinced Alpana, that she could also run this race. However, the conviction did not sink in Alpana for some time. Meanwhile, a new arrow was being honed to be added into her quiver of running in the form of Pinkathon.

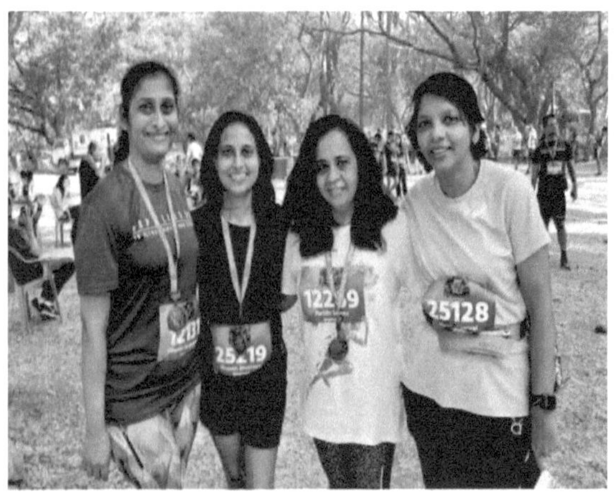

Runner Friends

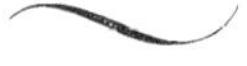

35

CHAPTER SIX

PINKATHON

"We all have dreams. But to make dreams come into reality, it takes an awful lot of determination, dedication, self-discipline, and effort."— **Jesse Owens**

Pinkathon is India's biggest all Women's Running Event. With Cancer Awareness as its associated goal, Pinkathon encourages women to adopt health and fitness in their daily lifestyles through running. Pinkathon is organized in several major cities of India and the number of women participants increases every year, a pointer that running as a sports event is emerging as a gender diffusion process.

In 2016, Alpana noticed registrations for PINKATHON advertised through the flyers. However, to her dismay, there were only two categories available for the runners to participate in 5km and 10 km. As Alpana was not keen on running either of that distances, she did not register. Though she did not register, she had a lurking doubt in her mind about the non-inclusion of the 21 km run as a part of the Pinkathon. She had heard quite a lot about Pinkathon on social media and was keen to be a part of it but sadly could not be a part of it in 2016.

Next year in 2017 again the same flyers for Pinkathon were distributed and as usual, the 21 km category was missing. Alpana was disheartened. Luckily, she met Blossom just a few days before the last date for registration. Alpana shared the disappointment of her category not being part of PINKATHON with Blossom when Blossom interjected and informed Alpana that it was very much there and she had already registered.

The 21 km run has a separate registration and one has to coordinate with the Pinkathon Ambassador for the half marathon. Based on Blossom's advice, Alpana could register for Pinkathon and the year 2017 ended with December run in the pink t-shirt. 2017 (Two Thousand Seventeen) ended on a high note with four runs in a year.

As one evolves through sports, one tries to search for variety and different flavours and this started happening with Alpana as well. She went for the 3.5 km Pinkathon midnight run on 29 Nov 2019, as she wanted to have a feel of running at midnight (normally running events all over the world happen during the daytime and this could be a rare instance of an event happening at night)! Her runner friend Renu Rajguru also registered for it. The venue at 11.30 in the night was a sea of women- women of all age groups had come from far-off suburbs of Mumbai to participate; some had even come with small babies. It was a remarkable sight. The place was throbbing with the energy and enthusiasm of women.

Alpana had planned that she would run at her usual pace. It was her first brush with a midnight running event and hence the apprehension. The start and finish point was Asiatic Library at Fort. Milind Soman (the actor, and model who is now the poster boy of Indian running space) flagged off the run at midnight. Alpana and her friend Renu were the last ones to start and Renu mentioned that they need to surge ahead or else they could get stuck with the slow runners running at the back.

As Alpana remembers: "Starting from Asiatic Library (Mumbai's iconic landmark) we passed across the Gateway of India. As we reached there, I looked to my right and saw the Taj Mahal hotel lit up beautifully in all its glory. We paused to click a selfie and continued running. Turning back from the Radio club, we came back to the starting point. It was a surreal feeling running on Mumbai roads well past midnight". It was a wonderful experience and because of Renu, the duo finished the run much earlier and for Alpana, it was her fastest 3.5 km run.

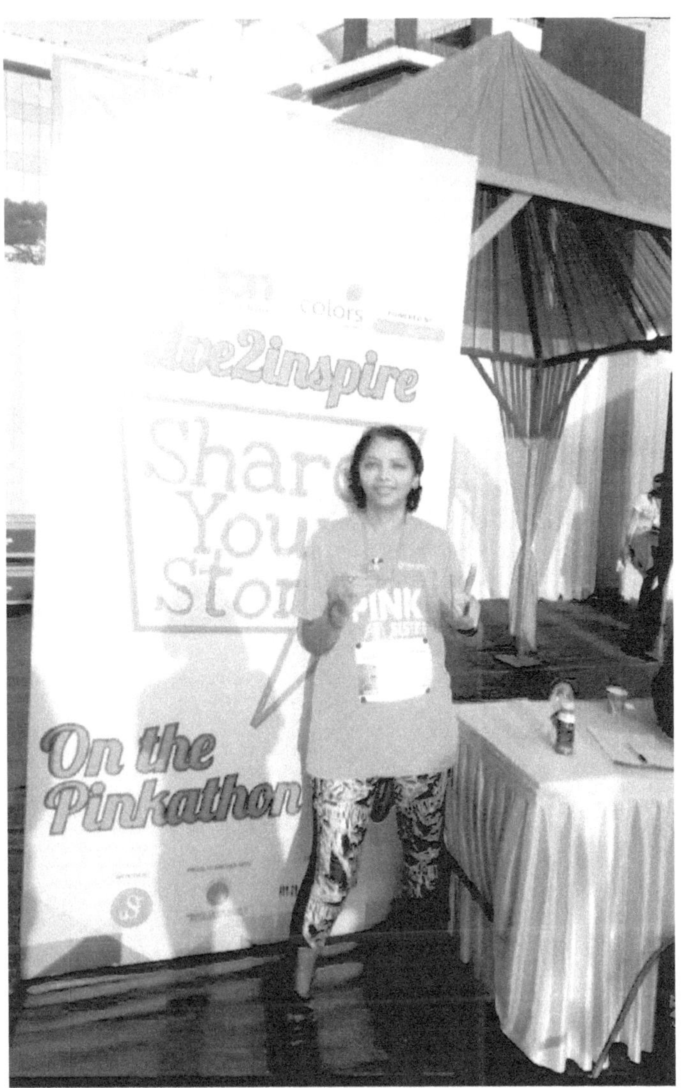

Pinkathon

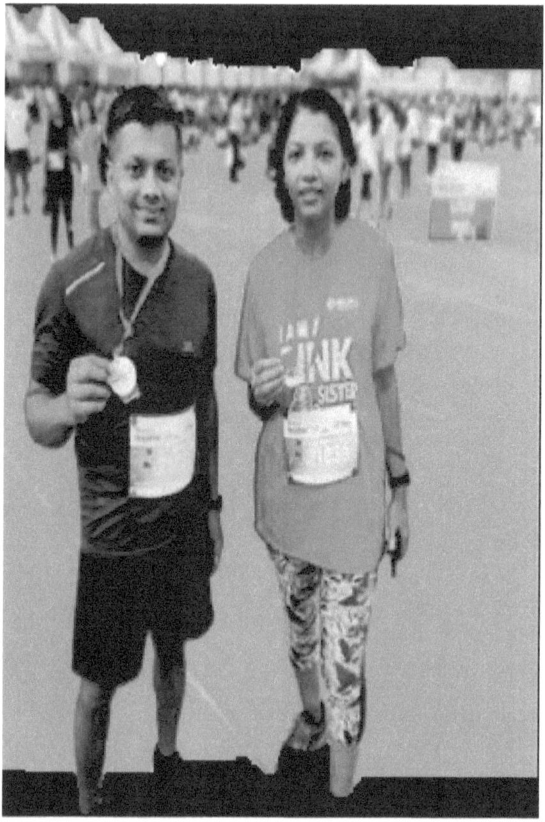

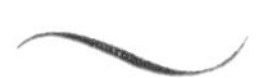

CHAPTER SEVEN

ROLE OF PACERS IN A RUN

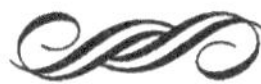

"We run when we're scared, we run when we're ecstatic, we run away from our problems and run around for a good time." — **Christopher McDougall**

All the marathons have pacers for different finish times and the job of a Pacer is to help the runners in his bus finish their run in the given time. Therefore, suppose you want to finish a half marathon in 2 hours but do not know how fast or slow to run to accomplish the task, a pacer helps facilitate it. He will help you run at a particular Pace and finish the run in 2hrs.

Alpana so far had no experience of running with a Pacer, as she preferred running at her own speed; slow, fast, or even walking if required. When she was planning to run the Navy Marathon, the organizers asked her to be a Pacer, as she had been a podium finisher and could be a good role model for the runners. Moreover, they were looking for only Navy personnel and their family members as Pacers, this being the Navy marathon.

For Alpana, this was a unique experience as she was going to be a role model for a bunch of runners and so far, she had not run a race herself with a pacer! The finish time of a pacer is decided after adding 15-20 minutes to the runner's personal best timing. Pacers are provided additional time so that he is under no pressure, run freely, are able to cheer up their fellow runners, take water breaks and finish the run comfortably.

Alpana's personal best time was 2.28 hours for a half marathon; accordingly, she was assigned the pacer ship and not the pacer bus of 2.50 hrs. *It was called a pacer ship as the Navy sails ships, and boats, and wanted to give a nautical theme to the event.* For the Navy marathon, pacer ships for 21.1 km started from 1.50 hours and with a difference of 10 minutes went up to three hrs. There were pacers for 10000m and 5000m runs. There were two pacers for each pacer bus.

For Alpana to be a motivator for other runners to finish the run, she had to calibrate her running timing. This being her first pacing, Alpana decided to run at an average pace of 7.5 – 8 km/hr to achieve the time of 2.50 hrs. This was a real test for Alpana as she had so far been running at her own pace, and now she had to set the tone of the pace for other runners!

A pacer can finish the run a minute before but not a second later than the finish time mentioned on the pacer's flag, a crucial point worth remembering while running. All the racers were given a t-shirt with their name printed on the back and their flags were handed over a day before the run.

Though she had to give up her own pace to enact the role of the pacer, she motivated fellow runners to finish off their races. It was a different experience for her, and the certificate of appreciation given by the organizers is a prized possession in her quiver.

After being a motivator and inspirer, now Alpana had to adapt herself to run with a pacer. She was apprehensive that the pacer might shadow her. So far, she had run all her races alone on her own at her own speed without a shadow! Her apprehension was that with a shadow running alongside, she might not be able to perform to the best of her natural ability.

However, these are mind games for sports where a sportsperson attains a comfort quotient with certain sets of combinations and one does not want to adopt, a dilemma that Alpana was also going through. Her doubts about running with a pacer were cleared, though, when she met her Pacer Mr Chetan Gusani. He was tandemly in a tango with Alpana's speed. The exchange of ideas while completing the process of running in the form of different running techniques engaged Alpana in conversation in such a seamless manner that she braced the finishing line without even realizing it.

A photographer by passion, Chetan is a software professional by vocation. He is present for almost every run/Marathon merrily clicking away pictures of the runners and it is a tough task. While a runner's job is finished after having braced the finishing line, a sports photographer has to be on his toes until the last runner has crossed the finish line.

Paying tribute to the undocumented efforts of photographers of the likes of Chetan, Alpana points out- "We runners shamelessly pester them for clicking our pictures in every possible running pose and they happily oblige us with a smiling face. Hats off to them for their dedication and perseverance". Chetan is just one of the tribes; there are others like Michael D'Souza and many more who tirelessly click pictures and motivate the runners to keep going. The mere sight of these shooters armed with their cameras brings a smile to every runner's face.

For her next **Pinkathon 18**, Sagar Bakshi was designated runner for Alpana. He had run the Mumbai full marathon and quelled many of her fears related to the upcoming 42.2 km run. He patiently answered all her queries and encouraged her to go ahead and conquer the full marathon! The pacer had paced the ambitions and through the pep talk had provided the launching pad for a full marathon.

Pinkathon's 2019 run of 21 km is another memorable run that was a milestone in Alpana's running oeuvre. The previous best record of Alpana's finish time for half marathons was 2.28 hours, and she had the innate desire to overhaul it. The process of overhaul did happen on 15th Dec.19. For this 21.1km run, her Pacer was Satish Kumar. As he was also from the Naval Community, Alpana knew him and had a quotient of comfort running alongside him.

At the starting point at Bandra Kurla Complex (the financial hub of Mumbai), Alpana shared with her pacer that she was a slow runner and expressed the desire to complete the run in around 2.30 hrs. Satish Kumar told Alpana that he was also a slow runner and would like to reach the finish line somewhere around 2.30 hours. However, as the run started he ran at a slightly faster pace than what Alpana had propositioned, but she was keeping pace with him. Satish slowly kept on pressing the pedal and both of them finished the race in 2.23 hours.

Her average pace that day was 6.45 min/km, while generally, her average pace is 7 min/km. Thanks to continuous motivation by Satish and cheering up by fellow runners; Alpana was able to achieve a new milestone.

However, she is not sure if this can be a new normal timing for her. Alpana aspires to run the Pinkathon in a saree someday.

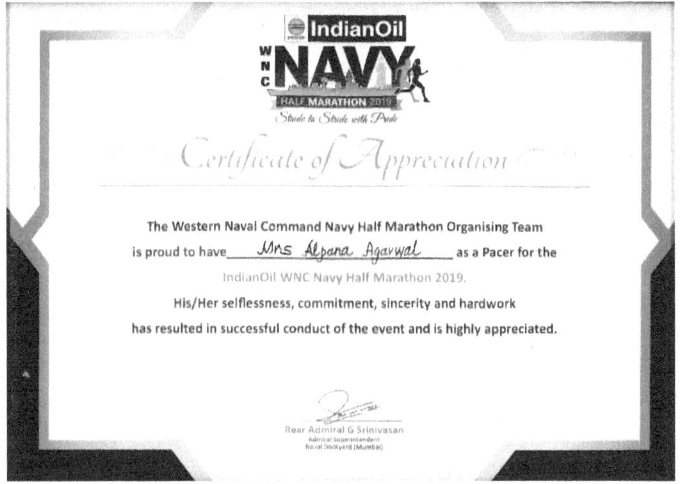

Navy Marathon

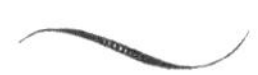

CHAPTER EIGHT

ULTRA MARATHON

*"If you are losing faith in human nature, go out and watch a marathon." – **Kathrine Switzer***

There are two types of ultramarathon events: those that cover a specified distance or route; and those that last for a predetermined period (with the winner covering the most distance in that time). The most common distances are 50 kilometres (31.07 mi), 100 kilometres (62.14 mi), 50 miles (80.47 km), and 100 miles (160.93 km), although many races have other distances. The International Association of Athletics Federations (IAAF), the world governing body of track and field recognizes the 100-kilometre distance as the official world record event. (Source Wikipedia).

Through Blossom- who had now become a new running friend, Alpana came to know that she had participated in a 60 km Ultra-Marathon. Alpana was awe stuck hearing the news, and though Blossom assured her that she could also run it, Alpana was not at all confident about running it.

On the face of it, there was a reluctance to attempt it, but the thought of giving it a shot had started germinating in her mind. When the idea generates, the second step is to start acquiring information about it and then test oneself, and Alpana set out on the quest to acquire the desired domain knowledge.

In the age of social media, even if the desired information may not come so succinctly, social media triggers the thought process through its tangentially associated posts. Alpana logged into the Facebook page of "Mumbai Ultra – the 12 hr. run" scheduled for August 2016 to gain knowledge on the Ultra-run. After going through it, she was convinced that it was an achievable task.

In Jan. 2018 after she ran 21.1 km in Tata Mumbai Marathon, the idea of going for ultra -marathon started taking shape. When she was convinced she could do it, she shared the thought with her husband and got a weird look as a reaction of not being in her senses! However, an Indian husband seldom disapproves of the idea proposed by a wife, so with a sheepish acknowledgement he concurred with the plan for the moment.

Alpana was contemplating running the full marathon (42.2 km) next year-(**2019**) and this appeared to be a good opportunity to test her strength and stamina and see if she could endure the punishing rigor of an ultra-marathon.

When February starts ending in Mumbai, the weather becomes hot and humid, and the end of February of 2018 was no different. In such weather, running even a few km becomes a punishment. Therefore, Alpana again hit the gym and this time her focus was on core strengthening exercises along with some weight training. As the days to register for Ultra run came closer, Alpana again discussed the topic of running the Ultra-Marathon with her husband.

He seemed worried that running this ultra-run might have an adverse effect on her health. However, Alpana convinced him that she had carefully considered all the aspects of the run and was confident about her strength and stamina. She needed her husband's moral support for her first ultra-run and seeing her determination he had no option but to support her and let her fulfil her desire of running this ultra-run.

In July 2018, she registered for the Mumbai ultra – 12 hr. run. Whenever she had butterflies in the stomach, she would call Blossom who had become her sounding board for Ultra Marathon. It was an endurance run and Alpana was certain that she would be able to do it. While the mind may be emitting intermittent signals of positivity, to convert the intermittent signals into a regular flow, it can only materialize when followed by physical preparedness as well! Alpana had not run for almost six months after a post 21 km run in SCMM (Standard Chartered Mumbai Marathon) in January 2018.

Therefore, she started running short distances every day. She was mentally prepared for it, but still, one day about three weeks before the run withdrawal systems crept in, she felt very low and underconfident.

As she reminisces about the final leap of faith "At about 3 PM in the afternoon I got up, laced up my running shoes and went out for a run. That day I ran 22 km in 3 hours and felt energized. The long run lifted up my sagging spirits and I felt I was ready to take on the challenge".

Mumbai ultra-run is a non-timed, run. Here one has 12 hrs. and you can run any distance which is more than 42.2 km. Basically, you have to keep moving, whether you run or walk, just keep going. You can rest if tired or advised by the medical team. It is an endurance run; you are relaxed and not under any pressure to finish the run within a stipulated time. There is no timing chip and no time limit.

15 August 2018 has a very special place in Alpana's life as on that day she clocked 60 km in the 12 hr. run. It was amongst her best runs so far. The motto of the run was "wellness over illness". The participants had to run or walk for 12 hours, from 5 AM to 5 PM. One had to keep moving.

Milind Soman's mother Mrs Usha Soman was also there and it was so heartening to see her walking with a smile on her face. She walked briskly throughout the day and kept encouraging other runners. Excellent arrangements by the organizers ensured the runners had a wonderful time. The route included running by the seaside at Worli Sea Face (one of the most famous promenades of Mumbai).

Crests and troughs of the sea waves, riding on the high tide at the peak of monsoon season leapt and lashed the seaside promenade. It was mesmerizing and forgetting to run. Alpana just stood there for a few minutes to soak in the beauty of the grey sea and imbibe the perambulations of the sea. The cascade of the waterfront at Worli Sea Face was an apt pictorial narrative of her preparation for the Ultra-Marathon, the lowering of her confidence and the final run.

Runners have to run in loops with each loop being about 12km in the Ultra-Marathon. Alpana ran the initial first two loops along with Blossom. Sharing the loop also fostered runners bonding.

From the third lap onwards, Alpana ran solo, as she wanted to cut down the pace of her running. Next two loops she jogged and walked. After the fourth loop, she had a light lunch. The fifth loop was completed by walking as she felt a muscle cramp in her left leg. By 3 PM, five loops were completed and she had covered 60 km.

After the fifth loop, she again met Blossom and Deo in the recovery area and veneered around to the view to call off running. (Deo is an enthusiastic runner and pacer from the naval community. He is always full of josh and motivates other runners to give their best).

Runners had a nice foot massage and a rejuvenating physiotherapy session. By now, it was almost 5 PM and all the runners were asked to assemble at the start point. As the clock struck 5 PM, the atmosphere suddenly became festive as all the runners congratulated each other for the successful completion of the ultra-run. All the runners were given finishers medals. A sumptuous dinner of Chole kulche and gulab jamun was served (perhaps to accumulate the calories burnt while running during the day).

Next year in Aug. 2019 The Mumbai Ultra run was again scheduled for 15 August. However, this Ultra run was hanging on the precipice as Alpana had registered for the Satara Hill Half Marathon to be held on 25 August. She was of the view that there would be less than 10-day gap for her to associate with Satara Marathon and decided to forgo this time.

Alpana turned around as she was motivated by the initiation of registrations for the ultra-Marathon by the members of her running group. She also jumped in and registered for the ultra-run. The run started with great enthusiasm and the first two loops were completed in a moment, pausing only for the mandatory medical checkup after the second loop.

The challenge started rearing its head from the third loop when monsoon showers soaked the runners and they were drenched from tip to toe. The socks were oozing with water, and though Alpana was carrying an extra pair of socks, she thought of changing them later.

She initiated her fourth loop of walking and then ran at a slow and comfortable pace to avoid any discomfort.

Monsoon showers reappeared during this loop and drenched the runners again. Alpana kept running in wet socks without pausing to change into a dry pair and it snowballed into a big mistake, which dawned on her when she entered the fifth loop.

Halfway into the fifth loop, she started feeling some discomfort in both shoes as if something was pinching the feet. Sitting at the Worli Promenade, she checked underneath her shoes but did not find anything, except for a particular spot on the sole of the left foot, which when touched, hurt badly, though, on the face of it, no blister had appeared on the foot. She did not pay attention to it and adorning the socks and shoes continued walking. When she reached the starting point, she went to consult a doctor for a medical checkup. The doctor informed her that due to continuous running in wet socks, sores had manifested and blisters would appear later. Alpana was not alone in this precarious situation, she found other runners also struggling with the same problem.

Doctor advised her to air her feet and rest for some time. Alpana started cursing herself for not changing the socks when they were drenched. The desi jugaad of putting some Vaseline on the exact spot in the feet, covering it with cotton and securing it with a bandage, she thought would help her, but she grimaced in pain when she put the foot down.

Clueless about the next course of action, Alpana found solace in her runner friend Aruna, who came to her after finishing another loop. Aruna advised her to put ice on her feet, have lunch and then begin again. It was 2 PM, with three more hours to go; Alpana was of the view that even if she walked slowly she would be able to finish the next loop.

However, the thought and the ground realities were different. Every step was adding to the pain quantitatively. A struggle between mind and heart started, while the heart was egging on to complete the race, the mind was giving signals to exercise precautions. Mind was giving signals of abundant precaution, as Alpana had registered to run for the Satara hill half marathon, which was barely ten days away. Eventually, the mind won over the heart and Alpana decided to call it off clocking 54 km.

She met her fellow runner Jatinder Deo, who too had stopped for the day after running five loops. He gave her wisdom on running by telling her that *they were not competing or running for others but only for themselves!* Hence, she called off her run at around 3 PM. On the day of the run, choices exercised are the best decision within the prevailing circumstances.

After taking this wise decision, she got her physiotherapy and foot massage done in the recovery zone. Later, she collected her medal, met all her runner friends, and pictures galore were clicked for posterity. Post a sumptuous dinner hosted for the runners by the organizers she headed back home as her husband and both her sons came to pick her up.

Within one year between the two ultras, she participated in IDBI Half Marathon on 30 Sept 2018. By now, she had convinced herself to go for a full Marathon and registered for the same with Tata Mumbai Marathon. The next month i.e. October 2018 went by without any long-distance run though she kept practising for the Navy Half Marathon to be held in November 2018.

Navy Half Marathon was successfully completed and in this edition, Ajay again ran 10km. The beginning of November brought along the news of a "Tribute Run" being organized to commemorate the 10th anniversary of the 26/11 Mumbai attacks. It was planned for 25 November just a week after Navy Marathon.

Alpana registered for 21 km here also and Ajay registered himself for 5km. When she told him about registrations he felt it was not advisable to run two half marathons within a gap of just one week. Alpana too realized her folly and mailed the organizers to change her race category from 21 km to 10 km. The organizers did not agree to her request.

Now she had two options. Either miss the run or go ahead and do it. Taking it as a practice run to check her stamina for the full marathon, she decided to run. As a backup plan, she had decided to walk if she found it difficult to run. However, all the fears vanished when she hit the track and she was delighted to finish the Tribute Run without any problem and within her usual time. The year 2018 ended on a happy note by running the 21 km Pinkathon. Though at the beginning of 2018, she was quite apprehensive about running two half marathons on two consecutive Sundays, now she doesn't even pause to think before running 21km on consecutive Sundays and does it regularly with élan.

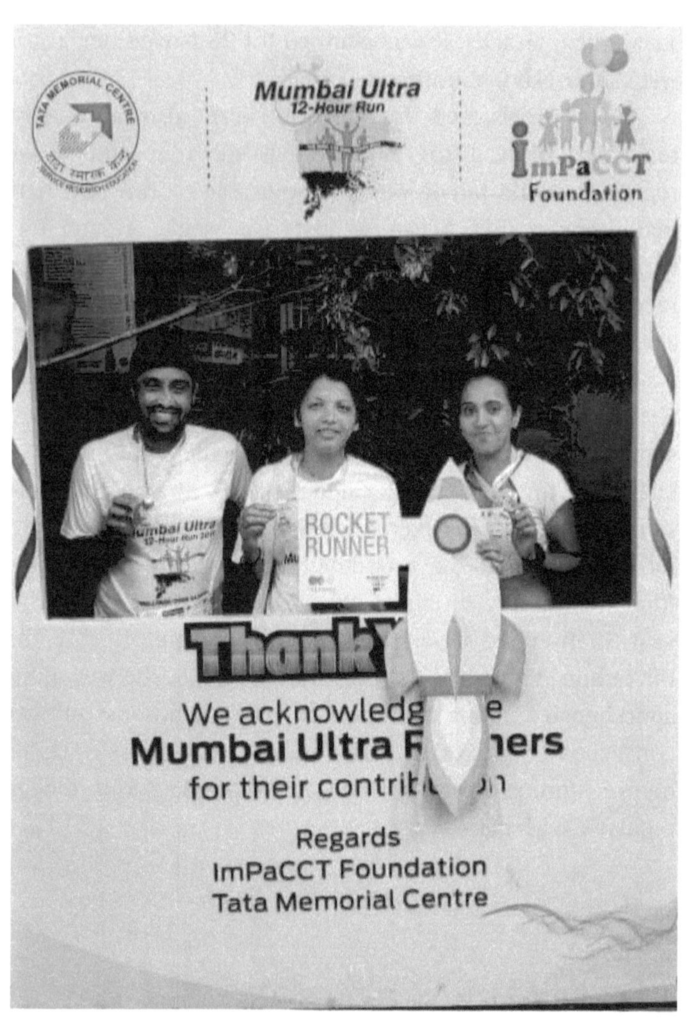

Mumbai Ultra Certificate

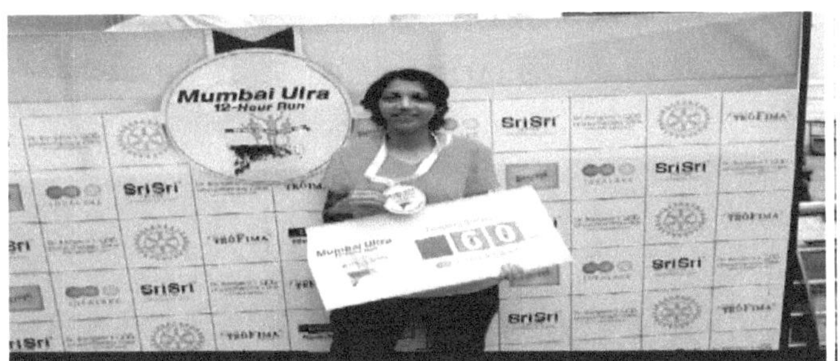

Mumbai Ulra
12-Hour Run
SriSri
SriSri
TRÓFIMA
SriSri
SriSri
SriSri

First Full Marathon·Run

"I always loved running…it was something you could do by yourself and under your own power. You could go in any direction, fast or slow as you wanted, fighting the wind if you felt like it, seeking out new sights just on the strength of your feet and the courage of your lungs." – **Jesse Owens**

The Marathon may have ancient roots, but the foot race's official length of 26.2 miles was not established until the 20th century. The first organized marathon was held in Athens at the 1896 Olympics, the start of the Games' modern era. The ancient games, which took place in Greece from around 776 B.C. to A.D. 393, never included such long-distance races. The idea for the modern marathon was inspired by the legend of an ancient Greek messenger who raced from the site of Marathon to Athens, a distance of about 40 kilometres or nearly 25 miles, with the news of an important Greek victory over an invading army of Persians in 490 B.C. After making his announcement, the exhausted messenger collapsed and died. To commemorate his dramatic run, the distance of the 1896 Olympic marathon was set at 40 kilometres (Source: History.com)

By now, Alpana had run 12 half-marathons and one ultra-marathon. She was quite convinced that the time was now ripe to go for a full marathon. After running Pinkathon in December 2018, Alpana took a 10 days family vacation to the North East and after coming back, she had three weeks to prepare for her maiden 42.2 km run before the Tata Mumbai marathon scheduled on 20 Jan 2019.

Experience shared by Marathon runners and the associated literature for Marathon runners advises a runner to go for a long run of 38km at least a month before the actual day. However, Alpana did not have that luxury as she was running half marathons back to back. Moreover, there was morbid fear of injuries during this practice run whereby she could miss out on the actual run, so she took to plan B to clock more than 42 km in a week.

Starting from 31 December 2018 to 6 January 2019, Alpana daily ran 6-7 km and clocked 43 km in that week. Satisfied with her efforts she took a break on 7 January and resumed the next day onward. On 9 January, a sore throat popped up but she ignored it as an aberration and continued to do practice runs. The morning of 10 January however came with ominous portents in the form of severe cough and fever.

With just 10 days left for the full marathon, Alpana was at her wit's end. She consulted the doctor and told her about the upcoming marathon. On the advice of her doctor, she took rest for 2-3 days along with the dose of medicine and then continued her practice as per her itinerary. As Alpana wanted her family to be there at the finishing line when her moment of glory arrived, she asked her son who was studying at Singapore to stay back and be at the finish line.

As the final day approached, she panicked. On the 19th morning, such was the nervousness that she almost cried with anxiety. Her husband convinced her that it was quite fine to be nervous; else, it would be a sign of overconfidence. Finally, the BIG day arrived!

As she glowingly rewinds the occasion-, "I came, I ran and I conquered the full Marathon. That moment when I crossed the finish line will always remain etched in my memory. The adrenalin rush, the excitement of reaching a milestone ...how I can ever forget that feeling of exhilaration and accomplishment after I completed my maiden full marathon in January this year! My husband and both sons were there to receive me after the run. As I collected my medal, I felt as if I was on top of the world. The euphoria of running 42.2 km just refused to die down. Everyone who came to know about my feat lauded my efforts, grit and determination, though most of them found it difficult to believe that I had run the full marathon. Nothing wrong, as I myself couldn't believe that I had done it".

Palm Beach Half Marathon On 7 July 2019 Alpana ran her next half marathon at Navi Mumbai. This run holds a special place in her life and will always remain close to her Heart. This time Blossom, Deo and Alpana all three ran together. Blossom was moving to Goa as her husband was under orders of transfer. This was going to be their last run together before Blossom shifted base. Therefore, she wanted to enjoy this run with her friends without bothering about the finish time. Alpana and Deo too decided to run along with her at her pace.

In Alpana's words, "Believe me, it was so much fun just running with friends and going with the flow. None of us even bothered to look at our watch and check the time or distance. We had a blast running this half marathon. We cracked jokes, pulled each other's legs, narrated anecdotes, and had a wonderful time running together. We ran slowly, walked several times in between and took much more time to cross the finish line than our usual time. Nevertheless, none of us had any qualms about our finish time. We wanted to enjoy the run and cherish the memories and surely, we did just that."

After this run, the next one was a trail run on 27 July 2019. However, the heavy rains that lashed Mumbai between 20th to 27 July 2019 flooded the entire area where the run was to be held. Keeping the safety of the runners in mind, the organizers postponed the run to 22 September. 2019.

Satara Hill Half Marathon

Mumbai Ultra Marathon having been done and dusted, it was now time to prepare for the Satara hill run. As a fall out of Mumbai ultra 12-hour run in August 2019, she had adornments as a memento in the form of blisters on both soles. The mind won over the physical infirmities. Within the next 2-3 days she had recovered completely and was eager to go for Satara.

Satara is a small hill station nestled in the Sahayadri range of mountains about 270 km from Mumbai. Satara Hill Half Marathon is an annual run in the historic city of Satara, the erstwhile capital of the Maratha kingdom founded by the legendary warrior King Shrimant Chhatrapati Shivaji Raje Bhosale. It is one of India's most popular and loved running events. It is ranked among the best in the world by **Distance Running Magazine** UK and is the holder of the Guinness World Records title for 'Most people in a single mountain run.

Alpana came to know about the Satara Hill Half Marathon through a runner friend who had done it in 2018. Alpana too was keen to take her level of running one notch up by running on a different terrain. This was Alpana's first outstation run in her running career.

Running Satara Hill Half Marathon, required preparation for hill running. Alpana started it in July and chose Malabar hill as the training ground. She could convince her husband Ajay also to come along and become her practice partner. The course marked out was from Chowpati, from then they would run up to the Malabar hill to Kamala Nehru Park, turn around and do one more upslope on the way and continue running till Marine Drive until the distance of 10 km was clocked. Climbing of steps was also included as a part of the preparation.

The apartment in Colaba where Alpana stays has 10 floors. She would walk up the ten floors and then come two floors down the stairs and take the elevator to reach the ground floor. She did this endurance exercise continuously for 45 minutes to an hour. The rigour of running and climbing stairs convinced Alpana that she would be able to conquer the hill marathon with ease.

Distance Running Magazine UK may have christened Satara Hill Half Marathon, as amongst the best in the world, but the ground realities are different. Satara being a small place, the organizers restrict the number of runners. It also has only two categories of runners-the local runners who are from Satara and the outstation runners. Local runners register before it is opened for other runners from different parts of the country.

Alpana's friends had warned her that this run was very popular and with a limited number of running spots available, the window to register is very short. The General category registrations started on 7 April at 5 AM.

Alpana's friends advised her to keep all the required documents at hand and log in a few minutes before the starting time. Now as luck would have it, the same day, i.e. on 7 April Alpana also had to go for "Run for Autism". Alpana asked her husband Ajay to do registration on her behalf. He did it dutifully, missing his weekly golf again. Even his golfer friends were surprised that he had to skip golf for marathon registration. All said and done he followed the instructions to the tee and secured registration for Alpana. The General registration category was sold out in 71 minutes, which was a new record for the organizers.

Satara Hill Half Marathon is also called Ultra Half Marathon because of its unique and challenging character. (Total elevation gain is 420m as the race progresses and culminates).

The run started at 6 AM sharp. The route had 8 km of uphill climb. The first 4 km was a gentle climb with flat terrain in between. The actual climb began at approximately 4.2 km as one approaches the Satara- Kaas road. It is the steepest climb of the route and generally, runners try negotiating it by walking and Alpana followed the same strategy. Maybe the walk has been chosen by the runners to negotiate this bend, as this particular stretch provides a panoramic view of Satara and its surrounding mountains on the valley side.

The climb ends at 7.75 km after which there are easier rolling hills, apart from some sudden surprise smaller hills along the way. When one has completed 10 km of run, one reaches the highest point of the route called Eagle nest point at an elevation of 1048m from the sea level. It follows the turnaround point. If going up is tough, coming down the slope is tougher. The steep slope downward demands a strategy to control speed or the momentum can roll the runner over. There are some spots on the track where walking should be the preferred option by the runner, or else there always is a chance that the runner may roll down the hill.

There are two categories of runners. One category of runners is those who associate with the run to get it ticked on their bucket list, but other categories like Alpana are those who are not interested or running after the target, but they want to run and brace the finish point, soak in the ambience and enjoy the occasion.

Alpana has had interesting encounters where her fellow runners get shocked when she discloses to them that she does not run for a target finish time but she runs to complete the laid-out track route. She runs and enjoys the process and takes it to the finishing line without bothering about the finish time, though she keeps a rough estimate of the finish time with herself and always finishes within that time.

Satara Marathon was her first brush with a daunting and treacherous climb, which only strengthened her resolve to complete the run. Fresh mountain air worked as an invigorator and she crossed the finishing line in 2.52 hr.

For small cities like Satara, occasions like Satara Marathon rejuvenate the whole city and the city is out in its finery to display the pride to the runners who congregate from all over the countryside and different nooks and corners of the world.

A participant in a sports event gets her rush of adrenalin from encouragement from the audience and inspiring music of thumping kind to motivate him or her to come out with their best performance. Events like running and cycling to an extent are perhaps one of the best options for the crowd to have a bird's eye view of the participants-a luxury which no other event provides around the world and this bonhomie and hospitality is what makes such events shining beacons in their respective categories.

Satara's popularity as an event also stems from the fact that during the race one can walk through a cloud, could be running under a scorching sun and could get drenched as well. Alpana experienced all of it during the process of running and came out shining ccolourscompleting her first Hill Marathon.

When she had decided to go for Satara Half Hill Marathon her husband Ajay and son Prakhar both opined that Alpana shouldn't run a Half Hill Marathon just 9 days after the ultra-run. However, in her heart of hearts , Alpana was convinced that she could pull it off. Therefore, she went ahead with her gut instinct and registered for the marathon. For Alpana, the Satara Half Hill Marathon run made her aware of her strength and capability and further strengthened her resolve and belief in herself.

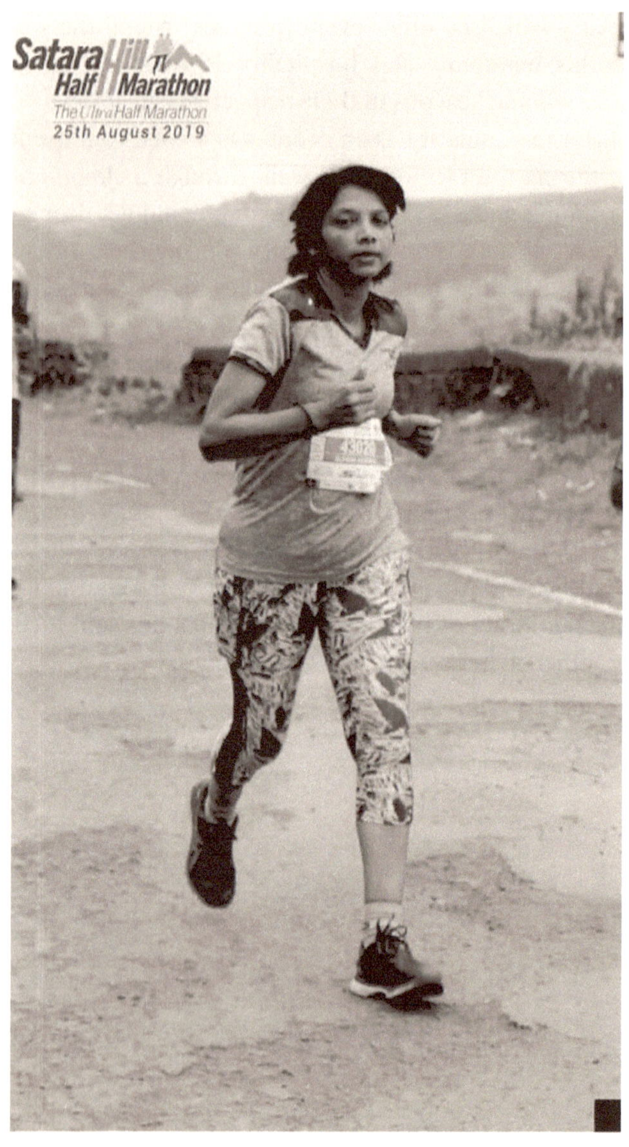

Satara Hill Marathon

<u>Alfa Run Challenge</u>: When you run a hill marathon, and that too a marathon of the likes of Satara Half Hill Marathon which is arguably one of the toughest, as a runner a feeling builds up that now you would be able to traverse such hill race events with relative ease. Alpana also developed this feeling after running the Satara marathon.

However, all her premonitions fell flat on the track when she decided to test her mettle in the Alfa Trail Challenge. This trail run was planned for 27 July. Incessant rains postponed the event. Now it was scheduled for 22 September. Though rains had reduced a lot in September, still two days before the run rains reappeared and a feeling of doom had started creeping inside Alpana.

However, as they say, the darkest hour brings the brightest light; it happened on the morning of the 22nd when the sun rose in its ssplendourbright and clear. Ajay had also registered for a 10km run as they both wanted to run on different terrain. The venue was at Rayate village near Kalyan in Maharashtra.

The start time for the 21km run was 7.30 AM and for the 10 km, it was 8 AM. By the time 21km started, it was quite warm. As it was Alpana's first trail run, Alpana had assumed that instead of running on the road they would run on a mud track. She however had no inkling of the strenuous route that lay ahead for her.

She was correct only to the extent that there would hardly be any road running. True to its name, the route was tough and challenging. Alfa trail Challenge had one of the most beautiful routes near Mumbai, going through mountain villages and scenic views of greenery and water bodies around. The trail run route passed through hills, paddy fields, streams and a wide tabletop plateau with flowering pastures.

The run traversed through a spacious wide terrain, a narrow single track, an exhilarating forest trail and a tricky muddy section. The route also had hill climbs with a 300 m ascent. The organizers had informed the runners that they should be on the lookout for red strips hanging on the bushes and branches to be sure that they are on the right track!

At some places, due to recent rains, the mud track was so slippery that it was a big challenge to even walk on it, leaving aside trying to run on it! Each step had to be traversed with abundant caution. As the route passed through tall grasses and paddy fields it was so quiet and peaceful that runners always had creeping doubt in their minds about whether they were on the right track at all.

However, the telltale signs of confirmation were in the form of red strips hanging on different street furniture on the landscape, and sighting them brought relief to the runners that they were on track. Along the route runners even had to wade through a water body that left the shoes soaked and heavy making it difficult to run in.

As the day progressed, the sun became brighter and all along the route, as there was no shade at all, the run became a test of endurance. The course of the track was studded with some admirable sights to ssavour but such was the luminosity of the sun that it did not allow the runners to stop and soak in the ambience

Alpana kept running and walking. The route was indeed beautiful but equally tough. Running on rolling hills on a mud track made the run very challenging.

This run would not have been a success without the angel volunteers who stood all along the route to help and guide the runners. Hats off to these selfless youngsters who braved the blazing sun with a smile. There were sufficient water stations with adequate water and energy drinks.

Running at a comfortable pace and walking when required she crossed the finish line and the cherry on the cake was a unique handmade medal (which has a pride of place in her medal collection). As it happened with the Satara Hill Marathon, local delicacies in the form of hot poha (local dish) and sooji sheera (semolina dish) were served to all the runners.

As a runner, Alpana has always gone for locally available food and has not yearned for protein diets or fashionable foods for supposed instant energy. She is of the view that our Indian food, after a hard and enduring run, not only satiates the senses but also plugs the gap for nutrients lost during the run.

The trail run gave memories in the form of badly tanned bodies, but full of memories of an unforgettable experience.

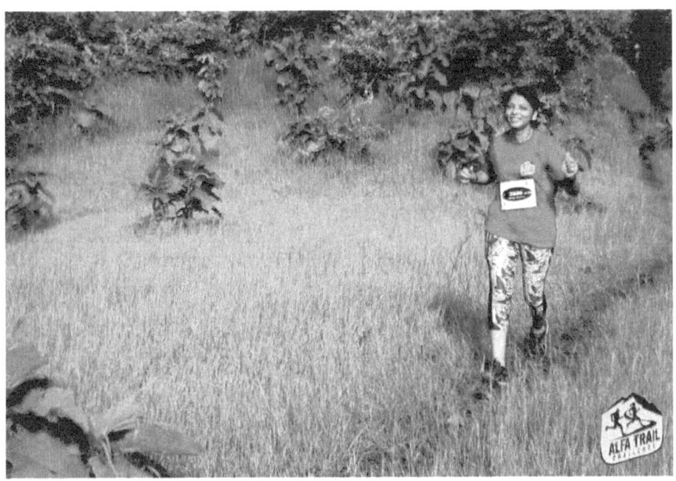

Alfa Trail

Borivali National Park Marathon (BNPM) And Other Runs

Having successfully run the full marathon, Alpana's next target was to run a marathon in changed surroundings. The opportunity came pretty soon when nature came calling for Borivali National Park Ultra 50.0 in Sanjay Gandhi National Park at Borivali, Mumbai. The marathon route included hill climbs. Runners could choose from three categories to run - 12.5 km, 25 km and 50 km.

Alpana registered for the 25 km marathon. This being her first hill climb marathon a sense of apprehension crept in. To prepare for an inclined run, she began her preparation by running on the incline runs on the treadmill.

The run was on 23 February 2019 a month after the full marathon. Her practice run on inclined slope in the gym helped her a lot on the race day. It was a pleasant day with a slight chill in the air early morning but as the run started, it became apparent that the route was tough, the roads were rough and hill climbs made it more challenging. The fresh air and pollution free surroundings energized her and she had a strong finish. Later in the day, it was informed to her that she had claimed the position of second runner up in her age category (female 51 yrs. and above). It was an occasion to celebrate, as it was her first 25 km run including hill climbs, that too just after a month of 42.2 km run and she was a podium finisher.

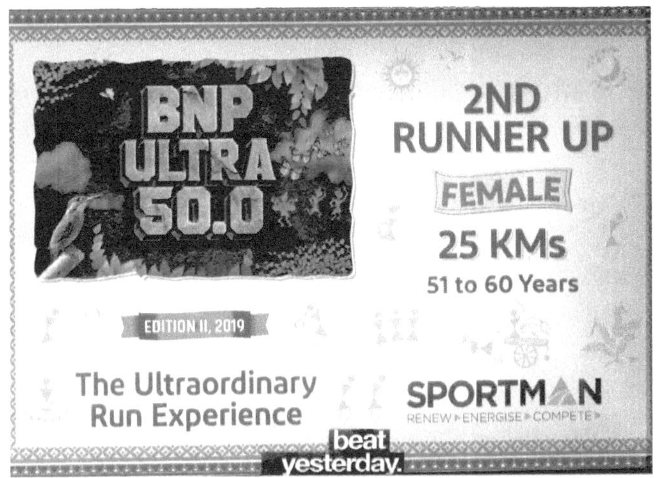

BNP Ultra Marathon

Second Podium Finish Within a Week: Just after a week of BNPM 25 km run Alpana found an announcement about the next half marathon-CANTHON (a run for cancer awareness) scheduled on 3 March 2019. Before registering for this one, she was in dual mind. The situation of two minds was that she was not sure if she should run another 21km just after a week of running 25 km with hill climbs.

Her friends suggested that she choose 10000m run if she was not confident. She veneered around the fact to run a half marathon, factoring in the premise that even otherwise, she had to get up at an unearthly hour and go to Dadar from Colaba, and there was no point relegating this effort to run only 10km.

As there was just a one-week gap between the two runs, Alpana went only for walks and did not do any strenuous exercise. The 3rd of March 2019 saw her all geared up for

Canthon. By now, she was brimming with confidence that she will have a good run. The weather was pleasant and the terrain was even. Her confidence in her ability to manage two marathons within two days culminated in her best timing so far!

She had completed 21 km in 2hr 28 min. In addition, she was again adjudged the second runner-up in her age category (female 46 yrs. and above). This was her second podium finish in a week. She did an encore on 7 April 2019 when she ran "the All in for Autism" half Marathon at Bandra, to obtain the podium finish of second runner up in the 45+ age category.

CHAPTER TEN

ROLE OF HUSBAND AND FAMILY AS A MOTIVATING FACTOR

*"Running became the one event in my daily life that I looked forward to. Books and movies paled in comparison to the refuge of my feet slapping patiently in the fresh morning air" – **Kate Kinsey***

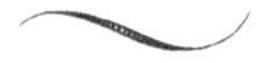

The saga with a run that began in March 2012, graduating from a daily run of 4 km to running a full marathon of 42.2 km in January 2019 has been interesting, though long journey. In these 10 years, Alpana ran 14 half marathons, one ultra of 60 km, one 25 km marathon and one full marathon. As she celebrated her 54th birthday on 21 August 2021, she was able to complete 54 runs for herself.

Her tryst would not have materialized but for the unflinching support from her family, more so her husband. In Alpana's case, the argument stands on its head- behind every successful man there is a woman, but behind this successful woman runner, there is her husband who often missed his game of golf to support his wife.

When Alpana had started running in 2012 in Navy Nagar quarters at Colaba, she had told her husband to keep an extra set of house keys and not wait for her after he came back from the office. Nevertheless, he would wait for her patiently to complete her practice and then both of them would walk together into the house. He was there for her first 10 km run, and also ran alongside her for moral support, though the race was to be run by women and he had invited amusing glances, but for Ajay to make Alpana a successful runner he bought all his might and support to the table.

When Alpana ran the Indore Marathon, he chaperoned her in his car cheering and motivating her. If he found a suitable place to park his car, he also ran a short distance along with her. When Alpana ran the half marathon in Indore, Ajay accompanied her to the venue and waited patiently for her to complete and then both went back together. Alpana found running as a bond of love to weave the family together into a solid unit.

After every marathon the moment Alpana lands home, she is greeted with a tall glass of fresh Nimboo paani (lemon juice). (What else can a runner ask for...!)?

After the Tata Mumbai full marathon, the finishers' medal that Alpana received actually had two medals, one for the finisher and the other for the inspiration medal for the person who inspired the runner. Her son was curious to know whose neck the inspiration medal should adorn. Initially, Alpana had this belief that she was her inspiration and nobody else deserved it. Now in the hindsight, however, she was of the view that if someone deserves that medal then it had to be her husband Ajay and she has gladly bestowed the inspiration medal upon him for supporting her. Her running saga has also inspired her family and now they are a runner family.

Other Motivators and Inspirers

While running as a profession may seem a lonely one, through sharing of experiences by competitors the process becomes fine-tuned. Alpana's evolution as a marathon runner has followed the same learning curve.

For Alpana, a suggestion from her husband's colleague- a seasoned marathon runner- to run at least one full marathon just for the experience, played an instrumental role in her journey to a full marathon. Suggestion by another runner to use energy gels while running for instant energy also helped in Alpana's evolution as a runner when she tried it for the first time in her ultra-run and full marathon and realized that it does give the runner a bolt of energy, which helps finish the run.

Alpana and her friend Blossom motivate and inspire each other to evolve as accomplished runners. Her casual tip to Alpana of having an early morning bath before leaving for a marathon, which Alpana had not adopted so far, changed her approach to running and made a significant difference in her overall demeanour.

Massage by a masseur is another tip from fellow runners that has helped Alpana in her running saga. The advice of the friends has been to have it two days before a run. She tried it for the first time two days before the Canthon Half Marathon on 7 March 2019. As she was trying it for the first time, she just began with the leg massage instead of the full body massage. She had an amazing podium finish and now massage is an essential part of her preparation for running any event.

Carb-loading and hydration is another mantra that Alpana adopted when her fellow runners told her about its benefits. Though she had read about carb loading on the internet, she had not followed it for her initial marathons. Carbohydrate loading or carb loading is a strategy used by marathon runners to maximize the storage of energy in the muscles. For the runner, two days prior to the race day you eat a high-fibre carbohydrate diet. Alpana had initially avoided this diet under the notion that she might add a few more kilos to her weight.

However, during the marathon running in the initial stages, she found her energy levels dipping just a few km into the run. Then she realized the value of carb loading. After adopting carb loading, her performance improved by a few notches.

Pre-marathon hydration is another facet that Alpana became aware of through a talk on marathon running organized by a runner friend. This also starts two days prior to the race day and involves hydrating yourself throughout the day. One has to increase the intake of fluids up to 9-10 glasses in a day. This is a sure shot method to avoid dehydration while running marathons, especially in the hot and humid weather of Mumbai.

Other than plain water, Nimboo paani, coconut water, fresh fruit juices without sugar and "enerzal" (a form of drink to prevent dehydration) can also be sipped at regular intervals. Following this hydrating technique, Alpana did not have the urge to have too many water breaks during the marathon which helped in saving up the running time.

Alpana now takes one break after 10-11 km and then stops only after the finish line

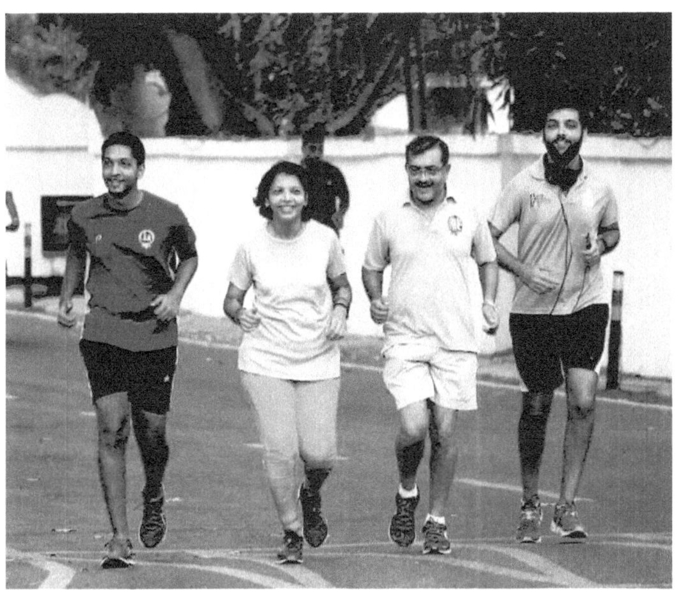

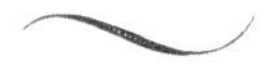

Family that runs together stays together

CHAPTER ELEVEN

SHEDDING SELF INHIBITION

*"I'm always nervous. If I weren't nervous, it would be weird. I get the same feeling at all the big races. It's part of the routine, and I accept it. It means I'm there and I'm ready."—**Allyson Felix***

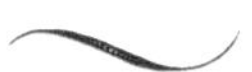

Alpana is one of those women who does not have a history of runners in the family and she is a self-made runner. One fine day just like Forrest Gump, she decided she had to run and she started running. While Forrest Gump did stop and wondered why at all he ran, Alpana continues to run and continues to experiment.

Navy Colony in Colaba- Mumbai has a stadium named- "Kohli Stadium" with a running track of 400 m. One fine day when Alpana had made up her mind, she landed at the track, with great apprehension and trepidation ran one round, and followed up with one round of walk and run again!

There was a perceived consciousness that Alpana was the focus of the eyeballs in the stadium, but then the realization dawned on her that everybody was busy focusing on their chosen activity and nobody was bothered about her. It was a shot in the arm for her confidence and in a matter of few days she was running ten rounds every day and it became her daily target. Some days, she would raise the bar and run 5 km as well!

From 4 km to 10km then 11km and then 21 km is how Alpana raised her racing bar. It was a slow transition. After starting a 4km run in March 2012, she ran her first half marathon in February 2015. During this period of 3 years, she was able to train her mind and body for the 21 km run.

It indeed is admirable to underline that whatever Alpana has achieved is without the help of a coach or through online running plans. For her first half Marathon, though she used the online training plans for reference. She also does not follow a structured diet plan, though she gave up on fast food and fried stuff ages ago!

She is an astute observer of fellow runners and clears quite a lot of her doubts with Google. Until the time she came back to Mumbai in 2015, Alpana was not a member of any runners group. As her friends gradually came to know that she was a long-distance runner, she was apprised of a runners group named "Sole2 Soul" and advised to join this group.

Most of the runners of her colony were members of this group. She was not keen to join it initially and declined the offer. During the next three years, she became aware of more such groups, but she chose not to take membership in either of them! She is a slow runner and wanted to be on her own. Later when she ran an ultra-marathon along with Blossom and Jatinder Deo (both members of the group), they were able to convince her of the benefits of being a member of the group and she eventually joined **Sole2soul.**

The best part of this association has been that now she is aware of all the information about marathons happening in and around Mumbai. Though she still runs alone, her participation in different Marathons has increased rapidly. One of the positive outcomes of becoming a member of the runner group was that now she could keep a tab on the various running events and register for them. Most of the time even bib numbers were collected by a group member on behalf of the runners. This saved quite a lot of time and effort.

When running a Marathon, Alpana believes in the mantra of not coming under any pressure and pushing herself, she runs as she enjoys running. Before the beginning of each run, she has a dialogue with herself that she will not go overboard and run at an uncomfortable speed. She also promises herself that the moment she feels she cannot run to the next step; she would start walking. She also aims to finish each of her races within the cut-off time.

The cut-off time for most of the half marathons is 3 hours and her target has been to finish it within that time. One can take more than 3 hours also but then timing mats and traffic regulations are removed, and once the traffic starts, it becomes difficult to run.

Alpana's priority is an injury-free and strong run. She detests the enquiry of fellow runners about her timing after the running event is over. If a runner has achieved her personal best times, she will broadcast it to the entire world and if she is not bragging about it then please do not ask about it at all.

She feels that the joy of finishing a run dissipates when people ask her about her finish time. She belongs to that breed of runner who is more concerned about enjoying the run and soaking in the sheer pleasure she gets while running. Therefore, she does not focus much on the finish time. Perhaps, subconsciously, a part of her wants to improve the finish time. However, she has realized that if she focuses on the finish time she is unable to enjoy her run. She is no more in the game of "pace race" and is satisfied with whatever time she takes to finish it. She is fully aware that being on the other side of 50, she cannot take any chances with her health by pounding and hitting it hard on the road. Moreover, she has been a podium finisher for a few half marathons in her age group while running at a comfortable pace, so she does not feel the need to push herself except for that last km when the finish line is visible and the adrenaline surges in her to give her best and embrace the finish line with aplomb. On the other side of the finish line, every runner is a winner, whether slow or fast it does not matter. We all run for our happiness and satisfaction, so each one to his own.

Alpana believes in her ability to finish the run within the cut-off time and more importantly have an injury-free run. She is quite gung ho about the fact that even after running a half marathon she still has the energy and stamina to perform her daily chores. For her running is over, when she crosses the finish line and after that, she returns to being a normal homemaker. She believes in the motive of running at a comfortable speed without sacrificing herself in any way in her daily routine.

The Zen state has dawned on her as she has seen it from very close quarters when runners overdo their runs and then suffer from serious consequences. She, therefore, exercises abundant precautions while running and never hesitates to walk or slow down as and when required.

The milestones of her running career are an outcome of the pace that she has adopted for her runs. She ran her first half marathon in 2015, and then took 4 years, 12 half marathons and one ultra-marathon to feel confident enough to go ahead for a full marathon.

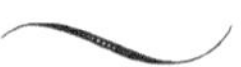

CHAPTER TWELVE

FITNESS IN PANDEMIC

"Your power has always lived within you...claim it."
Anonymous

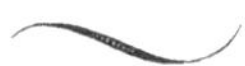

For runners like Alpana, who have gained momentum participating in different races around the country, when a lockdown is implemented and things come to a standstill, and you cannot move out, the abrupt halt in the momentum has a paralytic effect.

With no reference point in history to seek inspiration from and to tackle lockdown through the method of trial and error, trial owing to the initial stages of a scare against the unknown element of the pandemic and its ability to strike at will and without warning, and the error in sense of finding new ways to keep oneself fit!

For Alpana, the lockdown induced by the pandemic allowed her to look inwards and find out the storehouse of power hidden inside her body that she unleashed with a full vengeance taking out the stress and anxiety. Being a runner and used to running at least 5 days a week, the confinement within the four walls of the house was becoming claustrophobic.

They say necessity is the mother of invention and the lockdown induced an innovative approach to conjure up processes that would facilitate running. The passage in their house was the new track as it has a length of 13.5 m. Therefore, every day for about two months the family (Alpana's husband, two sons and Alpana) ran/ jogged the distance in loops for 30-40 minutes. This fitness routine through improvised running and focusing on core strengthening ensured that the family stayed fit and healthy during the lockdown and kept them away from any negative or depressing thoughts.

Alpana came to realise her real potential when she participated in a few online challenges during the Pandemic. First, one was a fitness challenge in a saree organized by Pinkathon Day Vizag on 28 April 2020. Participants had to do 10 push-ups, 10 lunges, 10 squats and a 30-sec plank in a saree and send the video to the organizers.

There was reluctance initially to undertake this challenge in a saree. Her family and friends motivated her and she went ahead and took the challenge. Alpana discovered that performing an exercise in a saree was not a difficult task at all. She came out as a triumphant winner in her age category of 50 yrs. and above.

A week later, the organizers came up with another challenge of doing squats for 30 min. in a format of 1-minute squats and 1-minute rest. The participants were free to do it in their way. It was held on 17 May 2020.

For Alpana, squats have been a part of her exercise routine for several years and she performs about 30-40 Squats almost every day. However, Squatting for 30 min.

seemed a bit challenging. Nevertheless, she went ahead with the challenge and recorded 790 Squats in 30 minutes. This boosted her morale and she realized that her body could take on such strenuous efforts also when there were no aches and pains after the Squats marathon.

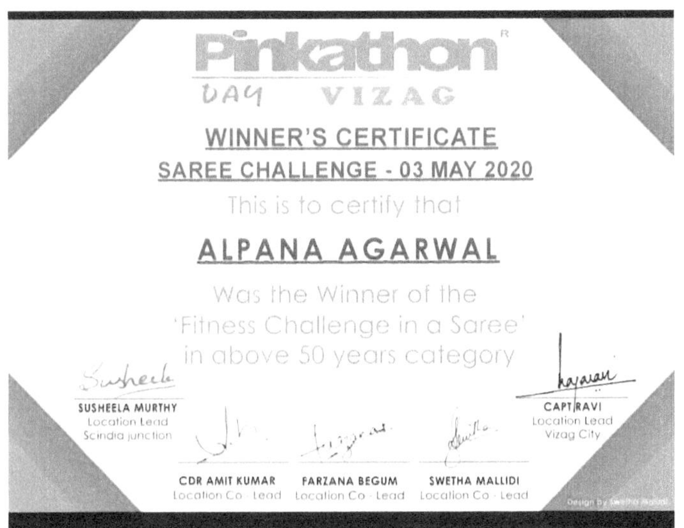

Saree fitness Challenge

Squat Marathon

Shortly, thereafter, through her runner's group, Alpana came to know about another online Squats Marathon scheduled on 30th May 2020 from 6.00-7.11 PM. Since she had already squatted for 30 minutes just a few days back she had the confidence to complete this Squat Marathon as well. The format was the same and within one hour and eleven minutes, she performed 2185 squats. For the event, 273 participants from 66 countries connected online and did 350,832 Squats to which she contributed 2185 Squats. It was a thrilling and an unforgettable experience for Alpana. Through this event, Alpana's faith in her inner strength was reaffirmed.

This Pandemic has indeed been a blessing in disguise. It has proved that human endurance has no boundaries.

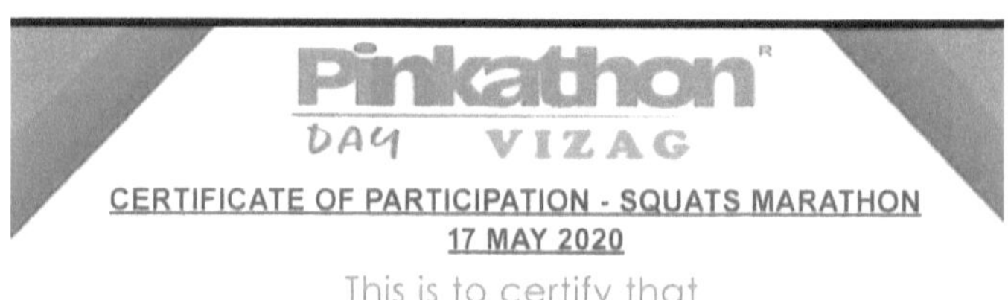

Squat Marathon

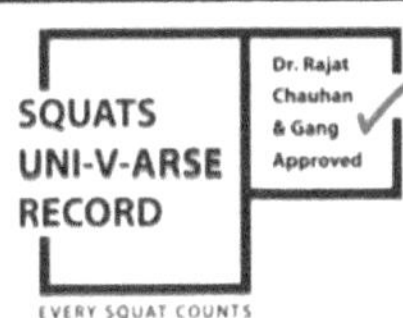

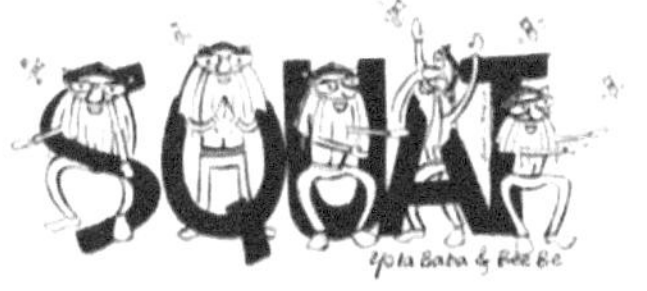

FAILING IS NOT A CRIME;

LACK OF EFFORT IS.

AND WHAT AN EFFORT IT WAS!

ON 30TH MAY 2020 FROM 5:55 PM TO 6:66 PM IST
273 PARTICIPANTS FROM 66 CITIES DID
350,832 SQUATS WHEN TARGET WAS 555,555 SQUATS

Alpana Agarwal

DID 2185 SQUATS

CONGRATULATIONS ON AN EXTRAORDINARY EFFORT.

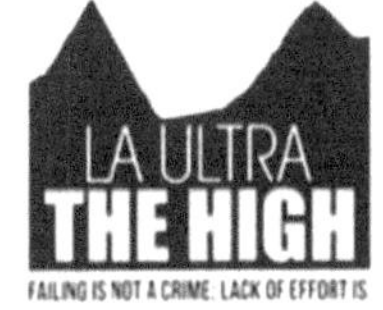

MoveMint
Medicine

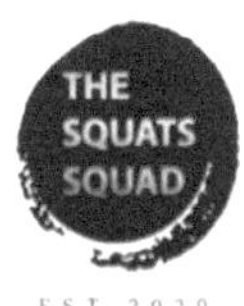

Squat Certificate

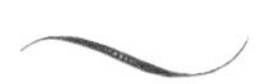

CHAPTER THIRTEEN

PREPARATION TO RUN

There will always be somebody more talented,
more beautiful, more successful.
You have to realize you're not running their race;
you are running your own race.
Joel Osteen (pintrest.com)

The milestones of success that Alpana has achieved in her running career have been without a full-time coach and guide. When she was making her debut for her first Half Marathon in Indore, her husband did suggest that she should train properly and systematically. However, Mhow, being a small town no facility for Marathon training was available. Therefore, she took preliminary help from Google and searched the net to have a general idea of Marathon training.

When she shifted to Mumbai, she dabbled with the idea of training under a coach but the timings and distances did not gel with her requirements. Even then, after having run so many marathons, she still aspires to train under a coach, to learn the proper scientific method of running and improve her posture. However, the moot point is, does she require it, after whatever she has attained in her running career so far?

The urge to run arose out of her determination to get back into shape when nothing else seemed to work and it was the last resort. Moreover, as they say, when you sincerely want something the whole universe conspires to fulfil your desire. Seeing the strides that Alpana was making on the running track, one of her husband's friends commented that even during his days as a young cadet in the Academy he did not run as much as Alpana was running!

It has been an exuberant and exhilarating journey so far. What began as a quest to initiate the process by running 4 km rose to 42 km and now it is 60 km. The trigger to graduate and evolve into a full marathon arrived while Alpana was running a half marathon and she saw the full marathoners happily covering the miles. The route of the Tata Mumbai Marathon is such that half and full-marathoners cross each other. While running her first half marathon in Mumbai in 2016 she crossed the full marathoners and was awe-inspired. In 2017 when she again crossed their path, her admiration for full-scale marathon runners evolved further as now she started looking at them with awe and admiration and wondered whether she would be able to follow their example and become a full-scale marathon runner.

In 2018, again, Alpana's paths crossed with the full marathon runners and she promised herself that she would become a full marathon runner so that somebody else may feel inspired and follow her. She promised herself that next year she would be amongst the runners whom she had been admiring for the last three years.

And the magic happened in the year 2019. A New Year and a new beginning, Alpana's dream was coming true as she was running her maiden full marathon on the other side of the road, which is allocated for full marathon runners.

She has a slight issue with her posture and while running she tends to look down- may be a by-product of avoiding the gaze, which sub-consciously became a part of her running style. This posture however started triggering pain in the neck and introduced a conscious effort on her part to look straight ahead during practice runs through this new adaptation, she has been able to mitigate the spasms of pain which had become an irritant feature of her marathon running.

She also has a bunion on her right toe; suffers from varicose veins that is part of her physical structure for the last 15 years. However, varicose veins troubled her, only when she was not running. Even the Bunion used to pain initially but then as with her continuous running, all the pains dissipated along with sweat.

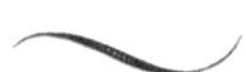

CHAPTER FOURTEEN

MIND RUNNING

Long distance running is 90 percent mental
and
the other half is physical – Rich Davis

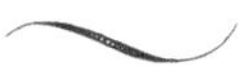

Sports Psychologist Garret Karmer in his book- Stillpower says that a key factor to performing well in sports (and in life), is your ability to control the quality and quantity of your "internal dialogue: understanding: Performance= Potential- Internal Interference. In other words, sports, business and indeed, life are played on a 6-inch course- the space between your ears!

Alpana is a mind runner. She runs with her mind. For her, physical training is important, but more than that, it is mental training, which works as a catalyst for her. She believes in the motto I CAN DO IT AND I WILL DO IT.

Before any marathon run, she starts preparing herself mentally. The process of mental training starts months before she actually starts her running practice. For the 12-hour run and the full marathon, she starts mentally preparing herself more than six months before she registers and started her practice runs. Mental training is nothing but believing in yourself, having full faith in your capabilities and adopting a positive approach towards your goal.

Human mind is very powerful. When you train your body to listen to your mind, together they can do wonders. She continuously reminds herself repeatedly that she can do it. She does not have the other option of not being able to do it. Once she has made up her mind to run a Marathon then there is no looking back. It is her positive thinking and firm belief in herself "that I can Do it ", is what keeps her going and helps her conquer marathons. It is indeed the conditioning of her mind to control the body that at such an age (50+) she continues to have her runs without any lay-off arising out of injuries of any kind.

Running after all is a mind game. As every runner says, 'It's all in the mind". Most ultras and full marathons are executed in conjunction with the mind. After some distance, your body may give up but if you have trained your mind well you will definitely cross the finish line.

During the initial half marathons after about 15 km, she had the incidences of withdrawal symptoms and negative thoughts of the likes – why at all was she doing this would swarm her thinking space. She would take a decision not to run again, but as the last mile of the finishing line would appear on the horizon, a positive adrenalin rush engulfs her to give her best and conquer the finishing line.

When Alpana decided to go for her first full marathon in January 2019, seasoned runners who had run 42.2 km warned her to beware of such negative thoughts. She was forewarned that after about 35 km negativity starts setting in as the runner reaches the killer incline of Peddar Road. One is already exhausted after 35km and on top of that, this incline really demotivates most of the runners.

For Alpana, however, this withdrawal symptom never reared its head as she reached the incline of the Pedder Road in her first full marathon as she had mentally prepared herself not to allow any negative thoughts to creep in and dissuade her from conquering the finishing line.

By the time one reaches Marine drive, the last 3km long stretch from there to the finish point is bereft of any trees and slow runners like Alpana have to run in bright sun. In fact, a runner later told her that after reaching Marine drive he was so disgusted that he actually wanted to quit the race and head back home (eventually, he did complete the run).

Alpana however emphatically rewinds to inform that throughout the entire stretch of 42.2 km, not even a single negative thought could rear its head in her mind. She crossed the Pedder road incline walking and jogging. Until the end, she maintained a comfortable and steady pace, walked a few meters in between and resumed running and riding on her indomitable spirit ran her first Full Marathon with panache.

Some of her friends who run 5km regularly recently ran their first 10km this year in 2020. They did well and when they met later, they shared their experience with Alpana that it was fine until 6-7 km but then they get bored running 10 km and kept waiting for the finish line and told her that they did not have a clue how Alpana could manage to run **Full Marathon and ultra-marathon.**

For Alpana her ability to conquer race after race emanates from the fact that it is not only her body that is running, it is also her mind that works in tandem spinning its own web and sending signals out to the body to keep pushing.

The bottom line however is, that after the race is over if Alpana tries to rewind to see what tapestry the mind has woven, she draws a blank and only remembers the prayers and chanting mantras- mantras and chants indeed have a power in getting focused and Alpana's continued success is a mental manifestation of the same.

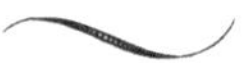

CHAPTER FIFTEEN

BATTLE OF BULGES

*"Weight loss doesn't begin in the gym with a dumbbell;
it starts in your head with a Decision." Toni Sorenson*

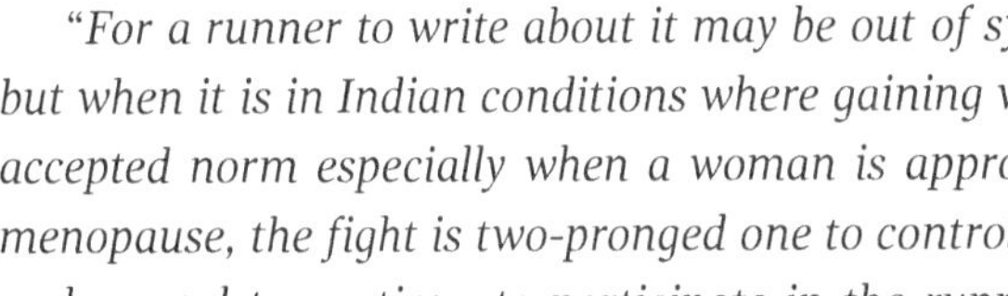

"For a runner to write about it may be out of sync usually, but when it is in Indian conditions where gaining weight is an accepted norm especially when a woman is approaching her menopause, the fight is two-pronged one to control the weight and second to continue to participate in the running events. To emphasize her struggle, this chapter is in the first person, i.e. Alpana herself remembering her struggles and triumphs. It makes it more so endearing as seldom a woman is candid to share her trial and tribulations to address weight gain issues more so when she is approaching menopause."

As mentioned earlier, my fitness regime and running helped me maintain a healthy weight for many years. However, the penny dropped a few years back when Mother Nature decided to step in and play her role. Yes, I entered the most dreadful phase of a woman's life..." Menopause". It began with a bang as bulges and curves aappeared left, right and Centre. For the next two years, my weight was on an uphill climb despite working out regularly and running half marathons. I was horrified to see my clothes getting tighter by the day.

For any social occasion where I had to wear a saree, it entailed detailed planning. I first had to check which blouse to pick up for alteration to gel with the occasion and with ease, and then the matching saree was picked up, rather than the other way around conventionally. Accordingly, Ajay was given strict instructions to inform me about any upcoming social event at least a week in advance.

The more weight gain, the more determined became my resolve to lose weight. It was a fight between the heart and the mind. I just could not accept this unfamiliar bloated figure. Heart said," it happens".

Every woman gains weight during menopause and you are no exception. Even my friends and family members very casually prompted me to accept it and not fight with nature. They tried to cheer me up by saying that you have enjoyed a healthy weight until now and a little increase in girth will not do any harm. One even mentioned that as you are taller than the average Indian woman is, some increase in the numbers on the weighing scale would not look so bad... (Pun intended) ...8 kg was just a slight increase!!!!

However, my mind simply refused to conform. I continued with my exercises and running but all my efforts seemed to be nought. In desperation, I convinced myself to visit the gynaecologist(I stay away from hospitals as much as possible) who promptly ordered a battery of tests especially, a thyroid test and confirmed that more than menopause slowing down of metabolism was the real culprit.

As it is with most children, I also had a severe needle phobia since childhood that continues until now when I am on the other side of 50. Just the sight of a needle drawing out phials of blood makes me feel giddy. However, Tests were conducted and the dutiful husband consented to come along just in case I ran away without giving my blood sample. (Yes, I have done this in my childhood and am quite capable of doing that now too). The results were normal and I was actually sad that I would not be able to blame my thyroid readings for the weight gain.

The option was to either sit and see myself ballooning up or get up and get going. As they say when the going gets tough, the tough get going. I gritted my teeth and braced myself to face this monster. Instead of getting demotivated, I continued running and exercising with vigour. In fact, I increased my running distance and the number of running days. Hard work always pays, though in my case the result came a little late. It was after about two years when the phase completely got over that I started noticing the difference. My old clothes started fitting better and the newer ones became loose. Inch loss was visible and I could finally fit into most of my old dresses. My active lifestyle ensured that I did not face any hot flashes, mood swings or depression, which are common during menopause and dreaded by every woman. It was smooth sailing for me largely.

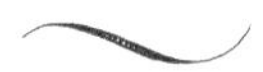

CHAPTER SIXTEEN

LEARNINGS

"Most people give up right before the big break comes —
<u>*don't let that person be you.*</u>*"*
Michael Boyle

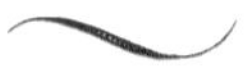

When you become an accomplished runner, you have trained your mind to perform as per the requirements. This control is accomplished by the choices of runs and Alpana in her running career has so far been very careful in choosing her runs wisely.

She aspires to run as long as she is alive and this is the investment plan that she is building up for herself. It is not easy to get up at 3.00 AM, leave the house by 4 AM and travel 20 – 30 km for running a Marathon. It is a commitment of passion to accomplish goals.

It is Alpana's innate desire that she and her husband Ajay should run a half marathon together someday.

The preference to run alone without a coach and immersed in self has its moorings in Alpana's determination to surmount the supposedly unachievable targets on her own. It was manifested in her routine sojourn over a flight of stairs up to an eighth-floor apartment, with her small son and his pram tucked along in Vizag.

From running for health and fitness to running for societal causes has been the trajectory that Alpana has traversed. The 12-Hour Mumbai Ultra run requires the runner to chip in with a donation towards the treatment of Pediatric Cancer patients at Tata Memorial Hospital, or the Canthon run to spread awareness about Cancer and build a cancer-free society or "All in for Autism"; running for such causes has brought out the humane side of Alpana. She now associates with such events frequently that contribute towards the betterment of a society or a segment through her sweat and grime.

She has also associated through technology via the "Impact" app. The impact is a corporate–funding, crowd-sweating, nonprofit-benefiting concept. This app helps raise Rs. 10 for a charity of the runner's choice with every km of walk/run covered on Impact.

As Alpana says: "Running has helped me come out of my comfort zone and achieve new milestones. I have learnt to believe in myself. The biggest lesson running has taught me is that nothing is impossible if your mind and heart are into it. Running has nothing to do with age. Age is just a number and that is what I firmly believe in. My aim is to run, run and run all my life."

Alpana is now wedded to running and lives the trials and tribulations associated with a wedding. She has her demons of burnout within a few years as she has now become addicted to running and wants to run two-half marathons every month. The lurking fear of burning out is simmering as she has seen this happen with a few of her runner friends who quit running either because of medical reasons or because they felt that they had too much of it. However, over the years, Alpana has gotten over her fear of burning out. Since September 2020, she has been on a running spree when Virtual Marathons became the new norm owing to the Pandemic.

Running in the Rain: In 2019, Tata Mumbai Marathon (TMM) started # "Mumkin hai campaign"- by Striders Miles, the official training partner for TMM to help runners prepare for the marathon. It was a three weeks free training programme before the actual run and Alpana also registered for it.

When Alpana landed on the first day of the training, she was the only runner present and it had started raining heavily. Alpana thought that the training would be cancelled, but the coach had different ideas. He asked her to run a short distance to check her posture and gait.

Imagine running in the rain at Marine drive and you are the only one running on the promenade. It was a heavenly feeling. That was her first run in the rain and now she makes it a point to run in the rain when it pours from the sky on the Marine Drive promenade. Her husband also joins in these rain runs.

Concerned about her poor posture which triggered neck pain while running full marathons, Alpana decided to find a solution to this problem herself. She worked on her own and was able to improve her posture.

Some of her fellow runners informed Alpana about three different types of training runs for marathons, namely, Tempo run, interval run and fartlek run. There is another variant to it known as the upslope run.

Tempo run

If your pace were seven, you would run at 7.5 or 7.3 for a chosen distance of the run. It is generally done during training and going for long runs and is generally done on weekends.

Interval training

Runner would run at his or her best speed for a chosen short distance such as 400/ 200 metres at the pace of 3 or 4, then walk and bring your heart rate back to normal and start again, a kind of start-stop method.

Fartlek

It is the advanced version of your interval training where you run for 300 meters at your best speed then to bring your heart rate back u do not walk but rather run only at a much lower speed. e.g., run for 300 meters at speed of 12 then jog at speed of eight or more. Generally, conditioned runners undertake this as it is a strenuous activity.

Running with husband

It seldom happens that when either of the pair is into one form of sports professionally, the other person follows suit. However, in Alpana's case, it has happened. Her husband from being the back office boy doing procedural formalities to smoothen Alpana's sojourn with the track has somewhere become a runner himself- though of a smaller magnitude. Ajay however has confined himself to a 10000 m run, though Alpana aspires that he graduates to 21000 meters so that they can run marathons together

The challenge for Alpana would come when her husband hangs his uniform and they shift base to National Capital Region (NCR). NCR climatically is in quite a contrast to Mumbai and she has the primordial fear that extreme weather conditions of the NCR may be obstacles in her running saga. The runner in Alpana however is hopeful that she would be able to find a solution to running in the extreme weather conditions of Delhi by the time they eventually move out of Mumbai.

Stadium run

For a runner, the bucket list is long and quite diversified. Throughout their running career, they strive to shift the bar and brace newer tapes. Alpana was no different, she had the secret desire to give a shot to Stadium Run- and she shared that it formed a part of her bucket list of runs that she had to accomplish in her running career.

A stadium run as the name goes is a running event to be executed within the closed enclosure of a stadium. Stadium run is of three different kinds- team relay run, 12-hour solo run and 24-hour solo run. It was Alpana's innate desire to be a part of a team relay run where a team of six runners is formed and each runner has to run for two hrs. Though Alpana has been running solo runs throughout her running career, she was not inclined to run a 12-hour solo run inside the stadium.

Running in a static landscape and orbiting it, as a satellite for 12 hours was not her cup of tea. The mere thought of it used to make her head go into a tailspin. In 2018 and 2019 her running friends had participated in the 12-hour relay stadium run but somehow she could not associate with it and missed it due to other commitments. However, in 2022 an opportunity to participate in 12 hr. stadium run came knocking at her door. She immediately grabbed it with both hands. To celebrate Azadi ka Amrit Mahotsva (75 years of Independence of the country) Western Naval Command organized a dawn to dusk stadium run from 6 PM on 19 March 2022 to 6 AM on 20 March 2022. The venue was her own backyard, the Kohli Stadium inside Navy Colony from where she had started her running career and it was indeed fortuitous that she would be ticking one of her favourite races from her bucket list as having scaled it.

From the time, the event was announced; Alpana was brimming with confidence that she would scale the 12-hour solo run. A recurring motif of Alpana's career has been the process of registration for an event, as registration becomes the trigger point to run in the event and is the motivation to participate in the event. To obviate an iota of dissuasion from inside, Alpana ensured that she was amongst the first few participants to register for the event.

Though Alpana in her zeal to tick her bucket list of runs had registered herself for the stadium run, she had to encounter two challenges associated with the event. First was that it was a night run from dusk to dawn. So far, Alpana had done two 12-hr runs but they were daytime runs from 5 AM to 5 PM. Then, the second challenge was running inside the stadium.

As a matter of practice, Alpana had done several runs for an hour or two inside the stadium and based on the laurels from the past she was of the view that she would be able to surmount the challenge of a 12-hour run as well! To be run ready (synonymous with the match ready), she ran a long run of 21km 10 days before the event. For the sake of acclimatization, Alpana executed her practice run inside the stadium in the evening and it induced the belief in herself that she would be able to complete the 12-hour run inside the stadium in that night.

12-hour solo runners have to undergo a mandatory health checkup before the event starts and subsequently every two hours during the run. The first check of the blood pressure before the run gave positive vibes to Alpana, as her blood pressure was normal. The run started sharp at 6 PM and Alpana began on the right note. B.P. was checked again after 2 hours at around 8 PM. All the vital stats were under control.

The weather was very warm and humid. She developed a cramp in her leg after running for about 25 km. After preventive medication, she decided to walk and jog. Dinner was served at 10 p.m. When the B.P. was checked for the third time, it was reported higher than normal. Alpana felt that the incidence of high BP could be because of dinner and she continued to run. She was asked to check her B.P. again. She continued to have a higher BP. Alpana did all stunts to bring it down, but the BP did not seem inclined to come back to normal. The doctor from the organizers' team strictly advised her to stop running.

Though there was no visible symptom of abnormal BP, the parameters arrived at through the clinical devices underlined the incidence of high BP. Therefore, Alpana decided to quit the race. The organizers were appreciative of her decision and gave her a participatory medal. Alpana however, refused to accept it. The organizers then informed her that she had fulfilled the criteria of being on the track for more than 6 hours, and therefore she had earned her medal. On being clarified that she indeed had completed the mandatory requirement, Alpana accepted her medal with graciousness.

With a medal in her hand and a sense of ennui about not being able to the most cherished item from her bucket list, she left the stadium run venue with tears in her eyes. She still could not believe that she had developed the symptoms of high BP and to affirm her conviction she checked her BP again at her home. It continued to be on the higher side. She accepted the fact that it indeed was a wise decision to quit the race and in her heart of hearts thanked the medical professionals associated with Stadium run to dissuade her from completing the run. Her BP stabilized in a day or two. However, to be on the safe side, for the next few days, she stopped running and instead preferred to go for long walks.

In hindsight, was it a failure that Alpana encountered in her running sojourn? Not likely. She tried something different for the first time and it did not work for her. Given an opportunity, she would like to go for this again and be better prepared this time. Bottom line is that every runner is aware of the fact that she has to listen to her body while running and act accordingly. For Alpana, through the rise in BP, her body was giving the signal that all was not well with her body and she had to rise to the occasion and heal the body before embarking on a new running mission. There was no point in associating with an event, which could open the door to hospitalization. Alpana throughout her running career has been in competition with herself and has given precedence to her health rather than tick-marking an event for record sake!

Alpana's running mantra is to remain injury free. She would continue to maintain the same until the day comes when she hangs her boots.

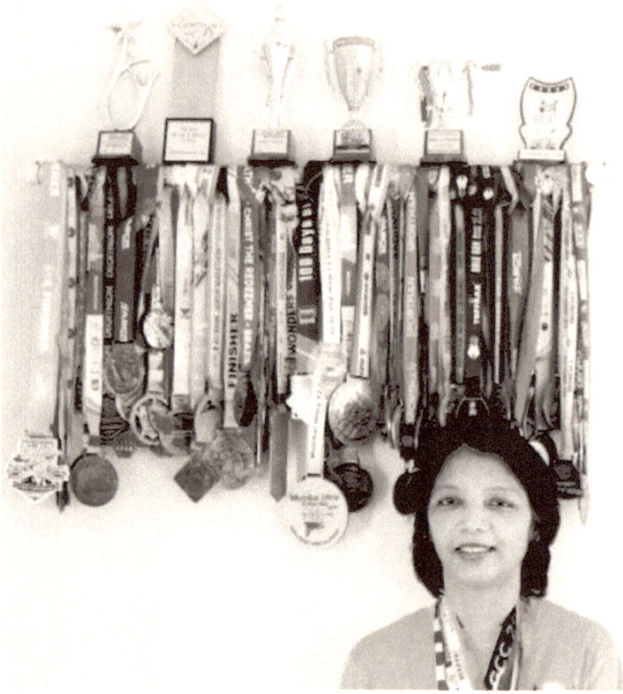

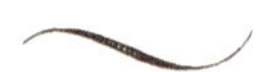

With the trophies collected so far

Epilogue

"I'll be happy if running and I can grow old together." –
Haruki Murakami

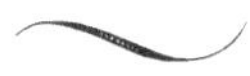

As outlined in the Prologue, when we had discussed this story, I had told Alpana that the world should read her story. She was reluctant initially, but later on, veneered around to the view that indeed this story has meat and it could become a source of inspiration for other fence sitters and reluctant runners.

The underlining premise of telling this story of Alpana is to make everyone especially women aware of the importance of physical activity in our life. She is quite confident that even if one of the readers, especially the women readers starts running or walking after reading it, the purpose of telling this story would be served to the T.

We ourselves are responsible for our health. One has to give a place of eminence to the role of physical activity in one's life. Alpana wishes to underline that by telling her story she wants to encourage the women folk to change their mindset and start giving equal precedence to self along with the needs of other family members.' The commitment to family is honed further when women look after their own health as when the woman's family head is healthy, only then can good care of the family be undertaken. Moreover, children emulate their parents, more so the mother. If the mother in the family leads a healthy and active lifestyle, the children too will be motivated and emulate the parents.

So instead of making excuses for not working out, think of ways to incorporate exercise into your daily routine. Actually, there is no need to take out extra time for exercise. If you cannot go out for a walk or run, exercise while working in the kitchen. Sounds impossible. However, it is easy, you only need strong willpower to do that or as Abdul Kalam, our President used to Say- I M POSSIBLE. One can easily do squats, on-the-spot jogging, and other simple exercises. While you are waiting for the milk to boil, do some lunges and toe touches. When you are on the mobile phone do not sit and talk. Make it a habit to walk inside the house while on the phone. Women folk are quite infamous for chatting for hours on the phone, chuckles Alpana, so why not turn it on its head and reap some benefit out of it. Keep walking and talking...it is that simple (provided the signals do not drop ☺).

After going through this story, if you feel motivated to run, then do not just go all guns blazing. Take it one step at a time. Start slowly by running short distances. You can walk and jog, say walk 100 m and run 200m. As your body gets used to running, increase your pace and distance. However, listen to your body. We are recreational runners and run only for our health and happiness. Each runner is different, so do not copy others. Do not compete with others; your only competition is with yourself. Set your own goals and challenges according to your capabilities and work to achieve them. Alpana set her own challenges and goals, worked towards them and was determined to achieve them within that time.

Over the years, Alpana reminisces that running has improved her posture and stamina and made her a positive person. The glow on her face has become a matter of discussion. In fact, one of her students in spoken English class, a young wife, one day asked her what cosmetic products did she use for the glow on her face. Cracking into a laugh, she unravelled that it was nothing but the consistent running she did that had contributed to this glow on her face.

People have different goals and aims. Most runners aim to improve their pace and achieve their desired timing. Her goal is different. She aspires to continue running until the last breath of her life. Pace and timing do not matter much. Her sole aim is to run and cross the finish line injury free. Her motto is "slow and steady". By following this strategy, she has managed to remain injury free until now and hopes to do so in future also.

With consistent running and regular workouts, she is at the stage where she can comfortably run 3-4 half marathons in a month. The month of March 2021, was very special for her. She had been planning to run half marathons on consecutive weekends for a month. She finally achieved this goal in March when she ran four half marathons on four consecutive Sundays. Not only that she also ran 10km on 8th March 2021, (Women's International Day) just the day after running a half marathon on 7th March 2021. The underlining part of this achievement is that she could do it with aplomb and panache without suffering any injuries at all. She is a powerhouse of stamina.

She often visualizes herself running happily down the years. Sh. Fauja Singh the oldest marathoner, who recently turned 111 years old on 1 April 2022, has been her inspiration and she aspires to emulate him. She is of the conviction that age is just a number and it is all in your mind. You are what you think. So, be positive, focus on your goals, work on your weakness and let your dedication change your personality.

The clarity of thought and sharpness of mind that ironically comes with physical fatigue.

The only boundary is what I set for myself and the only barrier is what I decide to break.

Running brings out the best of me and makes me more and more resilient to the challenges that life throws.

Who says it is a physical thing when all you need is a will and mind to push yourself? Legs just carry you across the line.

'The superwoman is CRAZY but TOUGH,

Like a SAVAGE, her FIERCE look brings out the warrior inside her,

She is BOLD, she is BRAVE,

She is like a diamond,

Tough and RESILIENT,

But always she is UNSTOPPABLE'